DECONSTRUCTING PSYCHOSIS

Refining the Research Agenda for DSM-V

T0176504

DECONSTRUCTING PSYCHOSIS

Refining the Research Agenda for DSM-V

Edited by

Carol A. Tamminga, M.D.
Paul J. Sirovatka, M.S.
Darrel A. Regier, M.D., M.P.H.
Jim van Os, M.D., Ph.D.

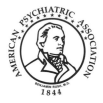

Published by the
American Psychiatric Association
Arlington, Virginia

Copyright © 2010 American Psychiatric Association
ALL RIGHTS RESERVED

Manufactured in the United States of America on acid-free paper
13   12   11   10   09   5   4   3   2   1
First Edition

Typeset in Adobe's Frutiger and AGaramond

American Psychiatric Association
1000 Wilson Boulevard
Arlington, VA 22209-3901
www.psych.org

Library of Congress Cataloging-in-Publication Data
Deconstructing psychosis : refining the research agenda for DSM-V / edited by Carol A. Tamminga ... [et al.].
     p. ; cm.
  Includes bibliographical references and index.
  ISBN 978-0-89042-653-1 (alk. paper)
  1. Psychoses. 2. Psychoses—Classification. 3. Diagnostic and statistical manual of mental disorders. I. Tamminga, Carol A.
[DNLM: 1. Diagnostic and statistical manual of mental disorders. 2. Psychotic Disorders—classification—Congresses. 3. Psychotic Disorders—diagnosis—Congresses. WM 200 D296 2010]
  RC512.D395 2010
  616.89—dc22

                                                                    2009005568

British Library Cataloguing in Publication Data
A CIP record is available from the British Library.

CONTENTS

CONTRIBUTORS

Jean Addington, Ph.D.
Professor, Department of Psychiatry, Faculty of Medicine, University of Toronto, Ontario, Canada

Judith Allardyce, M.D., M.P.H., Ph.D.
Senior Lecturer, Psychiatric Epidemiology, Department of Psychiatry and Neuropsychology, South Limberg Mental Health Research and Teaching Network, European Graduate School for Neuroscience, Maastricht University, Maastricht, The Netherlands

Francine M. Benes, M.D., Ph.D.
Director, Program in Structural and Molecular Neuroscience, McLean Hospital; Milliam P. and Henry B. Test Professor, Program in Neuroscience and Department of Psychiatry, Harvard Medical School, Boston, Massachusetts

Nick Craddock, Ph.D., FRCPsych
Professor of Psychiatry, MRC Centre for Neuropsychiatric Genetics and Genomics and Department of Psychological Medicine and Neurology, The School of Medicine, Cardiff University, Heath Park, Cardiff, United Kingdom

John M. Davis, M.D.
Gilman Professor of Psychiatry, Department of Psychiatry, University of Illinois at Chicago, Chicago, Illinois

Rina Dutta, MRCPsych
MRC Research Fellow and Honorary Specialist Registrar, Division of Psychological Medicine and Psychiatry, Institute of Psychiatry, King's College London, United Kingdom

Wayne S. Fenton, M.D.
Director, Division of Adult Translational Research, National Institute of Mental Health, Bethesda, Maryland

Wolfgang Gaebel, M.D.
Professor of Psychiatry, Department of Psychiatry and Psychotherapy, Heinrich-Heine-University, Rhineland State Clinics, Düsseldorf, Germany

Talya Greene, Ph.D.
Division of Psychological Medicine and Psychiatry, Institute of Psychiatry, King's College London, United Kingdom

Raquel E. Gur, M.D., Ph.D.
Director of Neuropsychiatry, Department of Psychiatry, University of Pennsylvania, Philadelphia, Pennsylvania

Assen Jablensky, M.D., D.M.S.C., FRCPsych, FRANZCP
Professor of Psychiatry, School of Psychiatry and Clinical Neurosciences, The University of Western Australia, Perth, Australia

Richard S.E. Keefe, Ph.D.
Professor of Psychiatry and Behavioral Sciences and Psychology, Department of Psychiatry and Behavioral Sciences, Duke University Medical Center, Durham, North Carolina

Jennifer Keller, Ph.D.
Senior Research Scholar, Department of Psychiatry and Behavioral Sciences, Stanford University School of Medicine, Stanford, California

Matcheri S. Keshavan, M.D.
Professor and Vice Chair, Department of Psychiatry, Beth Israel and Deaconess Medical Center, Harvard University, Boston, Massachusetts

Stephen M. Lawrie, M.D., FRCPsych
Professor of Psychiatry and Neuroimaging, Division of Psychiatry, University of Edinburgh, Scotland, United Kingdom

Mario Maj, M.D., Ph.D.
Full Professor and Chairman, Department of Psychiatry, University of Naples SUN, Naples, Italy

Kwame McKenzie, MRCPsych
Senior Scientist, Social Equity and Health Research Section; Deputy Director of Continuing and Community Care in the Schizophrenia Program; Professor, Department of Psychiatry, University of Toronto, Ontario, Canada

Robin M. Murray, M.D., D.Sc., MFRCPsych, FMedSci
Professor, Division of Psychological Medicine and Psychiatry, Institute of Psychiatry, King's College London, United Kingdom

Michael J. Owen, Ph.D., FRCPsych, FMedSci
Director and Head, MRC Centre for Neuropsychiatric Genetics and Genomics and Department of Psychological Medicine and Neurology, The School of Medicine, Cardiff University, Heath Park, Cardiff, United Kingdom

Mary L. Phillips, M.D., MRCPsych
Professor in Psychiatry and Director of Functional Neuroimaging in Emotional Disorders, Department of Psychiatry, Western Psychiatric Institute and Clinic, University of Pittsburgh, Pittsburgh, Pennsylvania; Professor of Clinical Affective Neuroscience and Honorary Consultant Psychiatrist, Department of Psychological Medicine, Cardiff University School of Medicine, Cardiff, United Kingdom; Visiting Professor in Psychiatry, Institute of Psychiatry, King's College London, United Kingdom

Michael Phillips, M.D., M.P.H.
Executive Director, Beijing Suicide Research and Prevention Center, Beijing, China; Professor, Departments of Psychiatry and Epidemiology, Columbia University, New York, New York

Darrel A. Regier, M.D., M.P.H.
Executive Director, American Psychiatric Institute for Research and Education; Director, Division of Research, American Psychiatric Association, Arlington, Virginia

Bruce J. Rounsaville, M.D.
Director, VA VISN1 Mental Illness Research Education and Clinical Center; Professor of Psychiatry, Yale University School of Medicine, West Haven, Connecticut

Alan F. Schatzberg, M.D.
Kenneth T. Norris, Jr. Professor and Chairman, Department of Psychiatry and Behavioral Sciences, Stanford University School of Medicine, Stanford, California

Carol A. Tamminga, M.D.
Professor and Interim Chair, Department of Psychiatry, University of Texas Southwestern Medical School, Dallas, Texas

Paul J. Sirovatka, M.S. (1947-2007)
Director, Research Policy Analysis, Division of Research and American Psychiatric Institute for Research and Education, American Psychiatric Association, Arlington, Virginia

Jim van Os, M.D., Ph.D.
Professor of Psychiatric Epidemiology, Department of Psychiatry and Neuropsychology, South Limburg Mental Health Research and Teaching Network, European Graduate School for Neuroscience, Maastricht University, Maastricht, The Netherlands; Division of Psychological Medicine, Institute of Psychiatry, London, England

Eduard Vieta, M.D., Ph.D.
Director, Bipolar Disorders Program, Institute of Neuroscience, University of Barcelona Hospital Clinic, IDIBAPS, ISCIII-RETIC RD06/011 (REM-TAP Network), Barcelona, Catalonia, Spain

Jurgen Zielasek, M.D.
Consultant Psychiatrist, Department of Psychiatry and Psychotherapy, Heinrich-Heine-University, Rhineland State Clinics, Düsseldorf, Germany

DISCLOSURE STATEMENT

The research conference series that produced this monograph was supported with funding from the U.S. National Institutes of Health (NIH) Grant U13 MH067855 (Principal Investigator: Darrel A. Regier, M.D., M.P.H.). The National Institute of Mental Health (NIMH), the National Institute on Drug Abuse (NIDA), and the National Institute on Alcohol Abuse and Alcoholism (NIAAA) jointly supported this cooperative research planning conference project. The conference series was not part of the official revision process for *Diagnostic and Statistical Manual of Mental Disorders,* 5th Edition (DSM-V), but rather was a separate, rigorous research planning initiative meant to inform revisions of psychiatric diagnostic classification systems. No private-industry sources provided funding for this research review.

Coordination and oversight of the overall research review, publicly titled "The Future of Psychiatric Diagnosis: Refining the Research Agenda," were provided by an Executive Steering Committee composed of representatives of the several entities that cooperatively sponsored the NIH-funded project. Members of the Executive Steering Committee included:

- *American Psychiatric Institute for Research and Education*—Darrel A. Regier, M.D., M.P.H. (P.I.), Michael B. First, M.D. (co-P.I.; consultant)
- *World Health Organization*—Benedetto Saraceno, M.D., and Norman Sartorius, M.D., Ph.D. (consultant)
- *National Institutes of Health*—Bruce Cuthbert, Ph.D., Wayne S. Fenton, M.D. (NIMH; consultant), Michael Kozak, Ph.D. (NIMH), Bridget F. Grant, Ph.D. (NIAAA), and Wilson M. Compton, M.D. (NIDA)
- NIMH grant project officers were Lisa Colpe, Ph.D., Karen H. Bourdon, M.A., and Mercedes Rubio, Ph.D.
- APIRE staff were William E. Narrow, M.D., M.P.H. (co-P.I.), Emily A. Kuhl, Ph.D., Maritza Rubio-Stipec, Sc.D. (consultant), Paul J. Sirovatka, M.S., Jennifer Shupinka, Erin Dalder-Alpher, Kristin Edwards, Leah Engel, Seung-Hee Hong, and Rocio Salvador

The following contributors to this book have indicated financial interests in or other affiliations with a commercial supporter, a manufacturer of a commercial product, a provider of a commercial service, a nongovernmental organization, and/or a government agency, as listed below:

Darrel A. Regier, M.D., M.P.H.—The author, as Executive Director of American Psychiatric Institute for Research and Education, oversees all federal and industry-sponsored research and research training grants in APIRE but receives no external salary funding or honoraria from any government or industry.

Nick Craddock, Ph.D., FRCPsych—The author has received grant support from the Wellcome Trust and the Medical Research Council.

Wolfgang Gaebel, M.D.—The author has received speakers fees from AstraZeneca. The author has received consultation fees from Janssen-Cilag, Lilly Deutschland, and Lundbeck Institute/Foundation.

Raquel E. Gur, M.D., Ph.D.—The author has received grant support from the National Institutes of Health (MH64045 and MH60722).

Assen Jablensky, M.D., DMSc, FRCPych, FRANZCP—The author has received research support from the National Health and Medical Research Council of Australia.

Richard S. E. Keefe, Ph.D.—The author has received research support from Eli Lilly and Pfizer through Duke University. The author is a consultant to Abbott, Acadia, BiolineRx, Bristol-Myers Squibb, Cephalon, Cortex, Dainippon Sumitomo Pharmaceuticals, Eli Lilly, Johnson & Johnson, Lundbeck, Memory Pharmaceuticals, Merck, NeuroSearch, Orexigen, Pfizer, Sanofi-Aventis, Shering-Plough, Wyeth, and Xenoport. The author is on the advisory board of Abbott, Eli Lilly, Memory Pharmaceuticals, NeuroSearch, Roche, and Sanofi-Aventis. The author has received unrestricted educational support from AstraZeneca. The author has received research support from Eli Lilly. The author has received speaker support from Eli Lilly. The author has received royalties from the Brief Assessment of Cognition and from the MATRICS Battery (BACS Symbol Coding).

Matcheri S. Keshavan, M.D.—The author has received grant support from the National Institutes of Health (MH64023 and MH45156).

Stephen M. Lawrie, M.D.—The author has received grant support from the Dr. Mortimer and Theresa Sackler Foundation.

Michael J. Owen, Ph.D., FRCPsych, FMedSci—The author has received grant support from the Wellcome Trust, GlaxoSmithKline, and the Medical Research Council.

Alan F. Schatzberg, M.D.—The author has received grant support from the Pritzker Foundation, the National Institutes of Health (MH50604), Bristol-Myers Squibb, Eli Lilly, GlaxoSmithKline, Somerset Pharmaceuticals, and Wyeth Pharmaceuticals. The author has served as a consultant to Abbott Laboratories, Aventis, BrainCells, Bristol-Myers Squibb, Corcept Therapeutics, Eli Lilly, Forest Pharmaceuticals, Inc., GlaxoSmithKline, Innapharma, Janssen, LP, Neuronetics, Organon Pharmaceuticals, Somerset Pharmaceuticals, and Wyeth Pharmaceuticals. The author is a founder and shareholder of Corcept Therapeutics.

Carol A. Tamminga, M.D.—The author has received funding from Acadia Pharmaceuticals, Inc.; Intracellular Therapies; Orexigen; Alexza Pharmaceuticals; Lundbeck, Inc.; the International Congress on Schizophrenia Research; the American Psychiatric Association; Finnegan, Henderson, Farabow, Garrett & Dunner, LLP; Synosia; Genactis, Inc.; and Astellas Pharma US, Inc.

Jim van Os, M.D., Ph.D.—The author has received grant support from or been a speaker for Eli Lily, BMS, Lundbeck, Organon, Janssen-Cilag, GlaxoSmith-Kline, AstraZeneca, Pfizer, and Servier.

Eduard Vieta, M.D., Ph.D.—The author has received grants and served as a consultant, advisor, or speaker for the following entities: AstraZeneca, Bristol-Myers Squibb, Eli Lilly, Forest Research Institute, GlaxoSmithKline, Janssen-Cilag, Jazz, Lundbeck, Novartis, Organon, Otsuka, Pfizer Inc, Sanofi-Aventis, Servier, Shering-Plough, the Spanish Ministry of Science and Innovation (CIBERSAM), the Stanley Medical Research Institute, and UBC.

The following contributors to this book do not have any conflicts of interest to disclose:

Jean Addington, Ph.D.
Judith Allardyce, M.D., M.P.H., Ph.D.
Francine M. Benes, M.D., Ph.D.
John M. Davis, M.D.
Rina Dutta, MRCPsych
Talya Greene, Ph.D.
Jennifer Keller, Ph.D.
Mario Maj, M.D., Ph.D.
Kwame McKenzie, MRCPsych
Robin M. Murray, M.D., DSc, FRCPsych, FMedSci
Mary L. Phillips, MRCPsych, M.D.
Michael R. Phillips, M.D., M.P.H.
Bruce J. Rounsaville, M.D.

FOREWORD

Rethinking Psychosis in DSM-V

Darrel A. Regier, M.D., M.P.H.

It is remarkable that the phenotype of psychosis that is standard throughout the world today originated in mid-19th century psychiatric hospitals with the formulations of Kraepelin. Now, more than 100 years later, this volume of papers presents a selection of papers reporting the proceedings of a conference titled "Deconstructing Psychosis." The conference was one in a series titled "The Future of Psychiatric Diagnosis: Refining the Research Agenda," convened by the American Psychiatric Association (APA) in collaboration with the World Health Organization (WHO) and the U.S. National Institutes of Health (NIH), with funding provided by the NIH. Summary reports from the other conferences can be found at the APA-sponsored Web site, www.dsm5.org.

Research Planning for DSM/ICD

The APA/WHO/NIH conference series represents a key element in a multiphase research review process designed to set the stage for the fifth revision of the *Diagnostic and Statistical Manual of Mental Disorders* (DSM-V). In its entirety, the project entails 11 work groups, each focused on a specific diagnostic topic or category, and two additional work groups dedicated to methodological considerations in nosology and classification.

Within the APA, the American Psychiatric Institute for Research and Education (APIRE), under the direction of the author (D.A.R.) holds lead responsibility for organizing and administering the diagnosis research planning conferences. Members of the Executive Steering Committee for the series include representatives of the WHO's Division of Mental Health and Prevention of Substance Abuse and of three NIH institutes that are jointly funding the project: the National Institute of Mental Health (NIMH), the National Institute on Drug Abuse (NIDA), and the National Institute on Alcohol Abuse and Alcoholism (NIAAA).

The APA published the fourth edition of DSM in 1994,[1] and a text revision in 2000.[2] Although DSM-V is not scheduled to appear until 2012, planning for the fifth revision began in 1999 with collaboration between APA andNIMH designed to stimulate research that would address key issues in psychiatric nosology. A first product of this joint venture was preparation of six white papers that proposed broad-brush recommendations for research in key areas; topics included developmental issues, gaps in the current classification, disability and impairment, neuroscience, nomenclature, and cross-cultural issues. Each team that developed a paper included at least one liaison member from NIMH, with the intent—largely realized—that these members would integrate many of the work groups' recommendations into NIMH research support programs. These white papers were published in *A Research Agenda for DSM-V*.[3] This volume more recently was followed by a second compilation of white papers[4] that outlined mental disorder diagnosis–related research needs in the areas of gender, infants and children, and geriatric populations.

As a second phase of planning, the APA leadership envisioned a series of international research planning conferences that would address specific diagnostic topics in greater depth, with conference proceedings serving as resource documents for groups involved in the official DSM-V revision process. In collaboration with colleagues at WHO, we developed a proposal for the cooperative research planning conference grant that NIMH awarded to APIRE in 2003, with substantial additional funding support from NIDA and NIAAA. The conferences funded under the grant are the basis for this monograph series.

The conferences that comprise the core activity of this second phase in the scientific review and planning for DSM-V have multiple objectives. One is to promote international collaboration among members of the scientific community, with the aim of eliminating the remaining disparities between DSM-V and the *International Classification of Diseases*[5] Mental and Behavioural Disorders section.[6] In January 2007, WHO launched the revision of ICD-10 that will lead to publication of the 11th edition in approximately 2014. A second goal is to stimulate the empirical research necessary to allow informed decision making regarding deficiencies identified in DSM-IV. A third is to facilitate the development of broadly agreed upon criteria that researchers worldwide may use in planning and conducting future research exploring the etiology and pathophysiology of mental disorders. Challenging as it is, this last objective reflects widespread agreement in the field that the well-established reliability and clinical utility of prior DSM classifications must be matched in the future by a renewed focus on the validity of diagnoses.

The APA attaches high priority to ensuring that information and research recommendations generated by each of the work groups are readily available to investigators who are concurrently updating other national and international classifications of mental and behavioral disorders. Moreover, given the vision of an ultimately unified international system for classifying mental disorders, members of the Executive Steering Committee have made strenuous efforts to realize the participation of investigators from all parts of the world in the project. Toward this end, each conference in the series had two co-chairs, drawn respectively from the United States and a country other than the United States; approximately half of the experts invited to each working conference were from outside the United States, and half of the conferences were being convened outside the United States.

A Broad Focus on Psychosis

The Deconstructing Psychosis research planning conference was designed, and the participant roster built, with the aim of reviewing an array of disorders in which psychotic phenomena are expressed: schizophrenia, schizoaffective disorder, bipolar disorder, major depressive disorder with psychotic features, and substance-induced psychosis. Logistical considerations precluded our expanding the conference agenda to other important areas, such as "functional" psychotic states seen in paranoia, psychoses associated with the dementias, and neurological illnesses such as Parkinson's and Huntington's diseases; clearly, however, it will be important in the future to more thoroughly compare the nature of psychotic phenomena, including localization of brain function, across these and other conditions.

This collection of papers is being published concurrently with the initial work of the DSM-V Task Force and its diagnosis-specific work groups. At the very least, the literature reviews and recommendations generated by our research planning conference participants will serve as resources for those charged with the revision; the extent to which the fifth edition of the manual—as well as ICD-11—ultimately embodies ideas and proposals contained in these papers will be a function of decisions to be made over the next several years, decisions that will incorporate into our current understanding of psychosis new information gleaned from research now under way. That said, it is timely to describe here the transition from the "planning" phase to the "action" phase of the DSM-V/ICD-11 revisions.

The conference agenda reflected continuing interest in the range of phenomenological manifestations that historically have represented our grasp of psychosis; these include but are not limited to delusions, hallucinations, cognitive impairment, family/genetic history, and culture-specific manifestations of psychosis. Additional features of psychosis are observed in other disorders. Psychosis associated with major depressive disorder, for example, is often characterized by neuropsychological impairments in areas such as attention, executive function, and verbal declarative memory. Beyond interest in knowledge gained to date, conference participants also looked ahead. During the research review, key issues emerged that cut across multiple diagnostic categories. These included interest in viewing and classifying mental disorders from a developmental perspective, reflecting a growing awareness that many conditions evolve over the life course. The notion of "disorder spectra" also drew attention across several of the planning work groups. Accumulating information about putative etiological as well as phenomenological features of different conditions raised questions about more informative approaches of "lumping and splitting" disorders in a manner optimally conducive to both clinical utility and future research. Spectra concepts might well also shed light on a necessary distinction between our current notions of comorbidity as opposed to a possible moderator effect of a given condition on another. Among the spectra considered during the review were those of psychotic phenomena associated with several disorders, obsessive-compulsive behaviors that may be common to multiple discrete diagnoses in the current classification, a new grouping of so-called stress and fear circuitry disorders that promise to reveal common neurobiological substrates, and the stew of generalized anxiety and major depressive disorders, to name a few. A third cross-cutting diagnosis common to consideration of diverse disorders concerns the somatic, or somatoform, features of mental illness, signaling widespread recognition that the brain is an organ much like—albeit at a greater level of complexity—other bodily organs; our understanding of mental disorders cannot be separated from broader health and medical concerns. Finally, and in large part due to the emphasis that the research review has placed on the demographic diversity and international representation of participants, attention to the influence of gender and culture on mental disorder has been prominent in our consideration of future mental disorder classifications.

Cutting across all of these superordinate topics is a mounting sense of the timeliness of incorporating dimensional approaches into our current categorical systems of diagnosis and classification. Long a topic of interest in the Axis II category of personality disorders, the question of dimensional approaches now has permeated thinking of traditional Axis I disorders. Indeed, the relevance of dimensional approaches to all mental disorder diagnoses and to promising endophenotypes of disorders prompted the addition of a work group/conference to focus on how dimensional constructs might be added to the classification in its entirety. Papers from that conference were published in July 2007 in the *International Journal of Methods in Psychiatric Research* and, like these papers on psychosis, became available in an APA monograph entitled *Dimensional Approaches in Diagnostic Classification: Refining the Research Agenda for DSM-V*.

As the formal DSM revision process ramped up in early 2007, the task force that coordinates the work of the diagnosis-specific work groups prepared working papers focused on these four topics, with the intent of setting a framework for the revision before the work groups became too deeply invested in a process of fine-tuning existing diagnoses.

We intend that the DSM revision work groups tasked with the array of disorders that subsume psychotic illness will carry forward the scientific reviews and open-minded thinking that characterized the research review process to more fully evaluate any need or potential benefits of proposing changes in definitions, boundaries, or linkages among psychotic disorders with other diagnostic domains in DSM-V.

It is clear to all of us that in the 21st century, the nosology of mental disorders will remain a moving target. With appreciation of the pace of progress in multiple areas, ranging from molecular genetics to brain imaging to social, behavioral, and anthropological science, we intend for DSM-V to be a "living document" that will explicitly be able to accommodate new research findings as they are replicated and are shown to better define and validate our diagnostic entities. That this will require a platform with greater flexibility than the one we currently use implies the urgent need to fully explore and take advantage of the similarly fast-evolving potential for electronic publishing and, in turn, continuous revisions of psychiatric classification systems in the decades ahead.

References

1. American Psychiatric Association. Diagnostic and Statistical Manual of Mental Disorders. 4th ed. Washington, DC: American Psychiatric Association; 1994.
2. American Psychiatric Association. Diagnostic and Statistical Manual of Mental Disorders. 4th ed, Text Revision. Washington, DC: American Psychiatric Association; 2000.
3. Kupfer DJ, First MB, Regier DA (eds). A Research Agenda for DSM-V. Washington, DC: American Psychiatric Association; 2002.
4. Narrow WN, First MB, Sirovatka P, Regier DA (eds). Age and Gender Considerations in Psychiatric Diagnosis: A Research Agenda for DSM-V. Washington, DC: American Psychiatric Association; 2007.
5. World Health Organization. International Statistical Classification of Diseases and Related Health Problems, 10th Revision. Geneva, Switzerland: World Health Organization; 1992.
6. World Health Organization. The ICD-10 Classification of Mental and Behavioural Disorders: Clinical Descriptions and Diagnostic Guidelines. Geneva, Switzerland: World Health Organization; 1992.

INTRODUCTION

Jim van Os, M.D., Ph.D.
Carol A. Tamminga, M.D.

Numerous diagnostic categories exist that can be used to order and summarize the various manifestations of psychosis. Although these categories are meant to refer to broadly defined psychopathological syndromes rather than biologically defined diseases that exist in nature, inevitably they undergo a process of reification and come to be perceived by many as natural disease entities, the diagnosis of which has absolute meaning in terms of causes, treatment, and outcome as well as required sampling frame for scientific research. Conceived originally to bring order and facilitate scientific progress, they were important in establishing communication about psychiatric entities. But they may also confuse the field by imposing arbitrary boundaries in genetic and treatment research and classifying patients into categories that upon closer examination have little to offer in terms of diagnostic specificity.

Given the fact that we have not yet discovered the natural boundaries of psychosis, but only observe its properties, the only way to achieve progress is to periodically reassess all the evidence in the hope of catching a glimpse of its natural pathology. This monograph is the result of such an endeavor and was carried out in the context of *Diagnostic and Statistical Manual of Mental Disorders* (DSM)-V. "Deconstructing Psychosis" was the fifth diagnosis-related research planning session convened under the conference series on the "Future of Psychiatric Diagnosis: Refining the Research Agenda" and was held at the American Psychiatric Association (APA) headquarters in Arlington, Virginia, on February 16 and 17, 2006. APA's American Psychiatric Institute for Research and Education sponsored the project in collaboration with the World Health Organization and the funding agency, the National Institutes of Health. The 5-year effort represents an unprec-

Reprinted with permission from van Os J, Tamminga C. "Deconstructing Psychosis." *Schizophrenia Bulletin* 2007; 33: 861–862.

edented scientific preparatory phase in advance of the next revision of DSM-V and other psychiatric classification systems.

A representative group of 21 scientists and clinicians from all over the world were approached with the task of helping to "deconstruct psychosis." They were asked to summarize the evidence from their respective fields relevant for the diagnosis of psychotic disorders, in particular with regard to syndromes currently referred to as schizophrenia, bipolar disorder, major depressive psychosis, and substance-induced psychosis. For each field, a presenter was asked to summarize the evidence, followed by an assessment of this evidence by a debater. Participants were asked to examine their respective fields for evidence regarding the natural occurrence of the psychosis phenotype, as well as evidence relevant for the validity and usefulness of diagnostic constructs.

The actual process of "deconstruction" was conceived as follows. First, the processing of scientific and clinical evidence was stratified by area comprising genetics, psychopathology, cognitive psychology and neuropsychology, epidemiology, neuroimaging, neuropharmacology, postmortem research, transcultural research, early intervention, developmental epidemiology, and addiction, with presenters and debaters in each field. Second, participants were encouraged to assess the evidence in relation to both categorical and dimensional representations of psychosis and in relation to both clinical and subclinical expressions of psychosis.

Because research with a specific focus on diagnosis per se currently is rare, the participants adopted the strategy of examining the general research evidence and making specific translations to diagnostic validity and diagnostic practice. For example, comparable neuroimaging studies have been conducted in bipolar disorder and schizophrenia, yielding suggestions of both similarities and divergence. While these findings regarding group differences are relevant with regard to the validity of diagnostic categories, they are a very long way from being relevant for the actual diagnostic process in a single patient. The aim of "Deconstructing Psychosis," therefore, was not to provide quick recommendations of which criteria to use for which categories in DSM-V. Rather, it attempted to assess to what degree current diagnostic practice is in agreement with data gathered in clinical and basic research; moreover, it intended to recommend which areas appear most promising for bridging the gap between current diagnostic practice and the natural phenotype of psychosis. It is hoped that the dissemination of this effort will contribute to more research in the area of diagnosis in psychotic disorders. Although our diagnostic classification systems are reliable and useful, they have limited validity in defining biological entities because these are unknown for most mental illnesses. This existence of diagnostic labels with limited validity in psychiatry needs to be tackled and improved with each subsequent version of our diagnostic systems.

1

DECONSTRUCTING PSYCHOSIS CONFERENCE FEBRUARY 2006

The Validity of Schizophrenia and Alternative Approaches to the Classification of Psychosis

Judith Allardyce, M.D., M.P.H., Ph.D.
Wolfgang Gaebel, M.D.
Jurgen Zielasek, M.D.
Jim van Os, M.D., Ph.D.

Worldwide, the *Diagnostic and Statistical Manual of Mental Disorders,* 4th Edition (DSM-IV)[1] definition of schizophrenia is the most influential in clinical practice and research.[2] Its clear criterion-based definition facilitates diagnostic agreement (reliability) and communication among practitioners, including comparable statistical reporting of incidence and prevalence rates.[3] It has high clinical utility, providing nontrivial information about course, outcome, and likely treatment response.[4,5] However, does this make schizophrenia a valid diagnostic construct?

Reprinted with permission from Allardyce J, Gaebel W, Zielasek J, van Os J. "Deconstructing Psychosis Conference February 2006: The Validity of Schizophrenia and Alternative Approaches to the Classification of Psychosis." *Schizophrenia Bulletin* 2007; 33: 863–867.

Clinical usefulness is embedded in the established criteria for nosological validation.[6–9] A diagnosis is considered useful if its antecedent, biological, social, prognostic, or treatment correlates provide substantial information not contained within the syndrome's definition.[7,10] If we accept this conflation of utility and validity, DSM-IV schizophrenia is indeed a robust construct, a model for conceptualizing complex clinical experience, guiding clinical management and predicting outcome.

Clinical utility, however, does not provide information about the fundamental nature and structure of schizophrenia; it does not answer the basic taxonic question "are the correlations of observed clinical characteristics, corroborative of underlying latent phenotypic dimensions (continuous distributions), latent categories (composed of one or more class or subdisorder, each with its own phenotypic presentation) or a mix of the two?"[11] That is, usefulness does not provide information on the construct validity of schizophrenia.[12] If our definition of schizophrenia does not represent a "real" construct in nature, then it will not delineate the true pathology and causal mechanisms underlying psychosis; it will obfuscate etiology. The developers of DSM-IV carefully point out that there is no assumption that each category is a discrete entity. However, they provide an operational definition of schizophrenia presenting the disorder as a condition qualitatively different from health (discontinuity between normality and schizophrenia) and qualitatively different from the other diagnoses (discontinuity between schizophrenia and the related diagnostic categories described in the classification system).

Below, we review the evidence for this and discuss alternative approaches to the classification of psychosis.

The Distribution of Psychosis in the General Population

Mounting evidence suggests that, in fact, there are no discrete breaks (demarcations) in the distribution of manifest (positive) symptom indicators of psychosis; delusions and hallucinations seem to have a continuous distribution in the general population.[13–25] Prevalence estimates, in nonclinical samples, range from 4%[13] to 17.5%[22] (with methodological differences likely to explain much of this variability), and results from a longitudinal study using the British National Psychiatric Morbidity Survey data found that 4.4% of the general population reported *incident* symptoms at 18-month follow-up.[25] These rates are not a reflection of unidentified cases "hidden" in the community because only a very small proportion of those reporting positive psychotic symptoms fulfilled diagnostic criteria for DSM nonaffective psychosis.[16,22]

How should we interpret this skewed continuum of positive psychotic symptoms? It may be an artifact, caused by measurement error; the use of lay interview or self-report methods may lower symptom recognition thresholds, so studies are measuring psychosis-like experiences, not necessarily related to the clinical features of a true latent category or disease entity. However, even if there is measurement variance between the symptoms elicited in the general population and those from clinical samples, this may be informative, given the fact that psychosis-like symptoms can be conceived as indicators of psychosis proneness, "clinical psychosis" emerging (with higher than expected probability) from the pool of those with psychotic-like features.[20,26–28]

The skewed continuum may be indicative of a latent continuous pathology in the general population. This is consistent with the prevailing view that schizophrenia has a multifactorial etiology where many different genes, which are neither necessary or sufficient causes, and of small effect, interact with each other and with environmental risk factors to cause the disorder, different combinations of risk factors resulting in a gradation of exposure and associated range of presentations from normal through to the clinical disorder. Published work supports this postulated continuity in the risk factor profiles for community-reported symptoms and schizophrenia, though much of the evidence comes from cross-sectional studies where the direction of the associations cannot be determined for exposures that vary over the life course. One study has suggested that there may be some differences in risk factor profiles for psychotic symptoms and clinical psychosis,[25] though this may in part be a consequence of using current urban residence as a proxy for urban birth and upbringing. If this finding is replicated, it would suggest discontinuity of risk factor profiles, though at a different point (threshold) on the indicator continuum than that suggested by the DSM-IV definition of schizophrenia.

These findings throw into doubt the assumption that schizophrenia exists as a discrete disease entity (categorical latent variable). The requisite population-based studies, using appropriate structural statistical analyses, e.g., finite mixture modeling (and its derivates)[29,30] or coherent cut kinetic methods[31] have not been carried out, so it is still possible that a dichotomous latent construct could underlie the skewed distribution of psychosis indicators.[11,32] The above approach uses delusions and hallucinations as indicators for the latent (continuous or categorical) construct schizophrenia. It remains possible that they are nothing more than epiphenomena or nonspecific surface symptoms, not core to the pathological process or perhaps even end-stage manifestations of schizophrenia.[33] If this is the case, then positive psychotic symptoms may not provide adequate coverage of the latent construct whether it exists as a category or dimension in nature.

Schizophrenia: A Disorder Distinct From Other Psychosis?

The symptoms used to characterize schizophrenia do not define a specific syndrome. Rather, the concept allows a number of different combinations so that many permutations of the defining symptoms are possible (i.e., it is a polythetic definition). These symptoms are also found commonly in the other categories of psychosis described in DSM-IV.[34] Recent studies using psychopathological dimensions (correlations of symptoms determined by factor analysis) suggest that the diagnostic entities are similar with regard to the key symptom dimensions of psychosis.[5,35–37] There is, however, variation in the dimensional profiles of different diagnostic categories in that individuals with a diagnosis of schizophrenia score higher in the positive, negative, and disorganized factors, while patients with affective diagnoses score higher in the manic and depressive dimensions and lower in the negative and positive dimensions.[5,38] This seems to suggest a quantitative variation in symptom dimension scores across current diagnostic categories rather than qualitative differences. The factor solutions across studies have been broadly consistent demonstrating a five-factor solution for psychosis—manic, depression, disorganized, positive, and negative (though there may be conflation of the disorganized and negative dimensions in first-onset samples),[39] reproducibility of this structure strengthens the findings. The true latent structure of psychopathology is still to be clarified, e.g., latent class analyses (LCAs) demonstrate similar indicator profiles to those determined by exploratory factor analysis (EFA),[40,41] confusing our understanding at the latent level. However, the overlapping co-occurrence of dimensions may be indicative of underlying shared risk factors, which are quantitatively rather than qualitatively distinct and continuously expressed. The ambiguous schizoaffective category may simply be the result of trying to demarcate, where in reality no latent discontinuity exists. Reasonable doubt exists about the true latent structure of the psychosis spectrum; therefore, the true appearance of psychosis in nature has yet to be determined.

Alternative Approaches to the Classification of Psychosis

REFINEMENT OF THE DIAGNOSTIC CATEGORY (SUBTYPING)

The clinical heterogeneity of DSM-IV schizophrenia could be reduced by refinement of the current definition, narrowing the concept, to describe more homogenous symptom clusters or subgroups.[42,43] One putative categorical subtype is the "deficit syndrome," characterized by enduring primary negative symptoms.[44] Association studies support the clinical usefulness of this subgroup[45–51] but tell us little about its construct validity. Does it truly exist in nature as a discrete disease entity (as its definition assumes) or are its observed associations with external validators the result of comparing high-scoring individuals with those scoring low on a latent (negative) dimension? If negative symptoms are associated with other important variables in the clinical, neurocognitive, social, or biological domain, any comparison of individuals high vs. those low in negative symptoms will yield significant group differences regardless of whether or not the true latent structure of negative symptoms is purely dimensional. A recently published study, using coherent cut kinetics, suggests that there may be a latent level discontinuity in negative symptoms within (chronic) schizophrenia, with an estimated base rate of 28%–36%.[52] The authors were unable to compare this empirically defined construct with that of deficit syndrome because they had not rated deficit symptoms in their sample. Further support for a possible discrete negative subcategory of schizophrenia comes from a study that used a surface data reduction method (principal components analysis [PCA]) to identify dimensions of psychopathology and found the negative factor scores were bimodally distributed in people with a diagnosis of schizophrenia.[5] If the PCA factor does represent a latent dimensional construct (which is not necessarily the case), then this suggests a quantitative discontinuity in the negative dimension.

An important limitation of this approach, however, is the use of chronic clinical samples because this can lead to artificial truncation of the symptom severity distribution, which can distort the results by violating the conditional independence assumption needed to obtain unbiased estimates.[31,53,54]

DIMENSIONAL REPRESENTATIONS

Another approach that has been used extensively to reduce the clinical heterogeneity seen in schizophrenia is by statistically identifying psychopathological dimensions (groups of symptoms that occur together more often than would be expected by chance alone) using factor analyses. Individuals can then be defined by how high or low they score on the different dimensions, which may coexist. This methodology assumes that the underlying latent structure of psychopathology is continuous. A three-factor solution has consistently been found in schizophrenia, and when affective symptoms are included, a further two factors are identified, namely depressive and mania/excitement.[55] Expanding this method to include more broadly defined functional psychosis has generally extracted similar four- or five-factor solutions.[39,56–59] Differential associations are consistently found across the symptom dimensions with clinically relevant variables.[5,36,38,60,61] Analyses comparing dimensional representations with the traditional diagnostic categories show the dimensions to be more useful at predicting clinical course and treatment needs, though the difference in the discriminative power may be rather small.[5,60,62] Thus, dimensions seem to add to the information contained within the diagnostic systems, providing assessments that are more detailed and likely to be important particularly in clinical research.

Both these alternative methods for classification (subtypes and dimensions) use latent variable modeling to tap into the underlying structure of psychopathology. However, the approach to date has important limitations. Taxonic analyses have rarely been carried out, prior to the LCA or EFA. Therefore, the decision about which statistical method to use has not been empirically driven but rather reflects the researcher's epistemological stance. If a latent class (taxon) is identified, external analyses (association studies) can be carried out on this subsample of individuals to determine secondary thresholds (subgroups). Failure to restrict these analyses to the taxonic group will introduce unnecessary imprecision into the search for secondary thresholds. On the other hand, if no taxon is identified, it is appropriate to use factor analyses or multidimensional scaling to generate symptom scores, which can be used in external (association) analyses to define diagnostic thresholds. It is important to remember that a latent class can be extracted as a strong factor in EFA.[31] Kessler has proposed a three-tiered approach for the use of structural analyses in the development of psychiatric classification systems.[53]

SEARCH FOR MORE PROXIMAL INDICATORS OF PSYCHOSIS

The current definition of schizophrenia and the alternative approaches discussed in this chapter depend heavily on symptoms and signs that are probably somewhat distal to the underlying pathoetiology. Integration of defining characteristics, more proximal to the pathological process underlying schizophrenia, is likely at some point in the future (reviewed in accompanying chapters in this book). Potentially informative, alternative indicators of psychopathology are the development of standardized and validated functional clinical tests for psychological dysfunction (dysfunctional modules).[63] A modular concept of psychopathology is grounded in experimental psychological theory, and depends on a model where psychological behavior and brain structure constitute a molar system, made up of identifiable microsubsystems of elementary psychological functions, with corresponding neuronal circuits, distributed networks,[64] or processing streams. A series or hierarchy of dysfunctional modules would then provide a detailed and individual characterization of an individual patient.

Conclusion/Recommendations

Two main diagnostic issues arise. First, it is essential to know how the psychosis phenotype or phenotypes exist in nature, in order to study its causes and outcomes. Second, a decision needs to be made about how to derive a useful diagnostic construct from the natural phenotype or phenotypes, so that patients can be usefully identified and treated.

In the short term, there is considerable need for descriptive and latent variable approaches to determine how psychosis is distributed in the general population. Identification of naturally occurring taxons, and/or continuous dimensional representations of psychopathology, and their associated course and outcome over time may be clinically very useful.

In the longer term, these descriptive approaches will no doubt be complemented by studies of putative etiological or pathophysiological indicators. However, until this time, the aim of any revision of our classification system should be to optimize clinical utility. The emerging evidence seems to demonstrate that models using both categorical and dimensional representations of psychosis are better discriminators of course and outcome than either model independently. Currently, the most useful approach to classification seems to be the complementary use of categorical and dimensional representations of psychosis.

References

1. American Psychiatric Association. Diagnostic and Statistical Manual of Mental Disorders. 4th ed. Washington, DC: American Psychiatric Association; 1994.
2. Mezzich JE. International surveys on the use of ICD-10 and related diagnostic systems. Psychopathology. 2002;35:72–75.
3. Kendell R, Jablensky A. Distinguishing between the validity and the utility of psychiatric diagnoses. Am J Psychiatry. 2003;160:4–12.
4. Bromet EJ, Naz B, Fochtmann LJ, Carlson GA, Tanenberg-Karant M. Long-term diagnostic stability and outcome in recent first-episode cohort studies of schizophrenia. Schizophr Bull. 2005;31:639–649.
5. Dikeos DGM, Wickham HMMF, McDonald CMMP, et al. Distribution of symptom dimensions across Kraepelinian divisions. Br J Psychiatry. 2006;189:346–353.
6. Andreasen NC. The validation of psychiatric diagnosis: new models and approaches. Am J Psychiatry. 1995;152:161–162.
7. Kendell RE. Clinical validity. Psychol Med. 1989;19:45–55.
8. Kendler KS. The nosologic validity of paranoia (simple delusional disorder). A review. Arch Gen Psychiatry. 1980;37:699–706.
9. Robins E, Guze SB. Establishment of diagnostic validity in psychiatric illness: its application to schizophrenia. Am J Psychiatry. 1970;126:983–987.
10. Spitzer RL. Values and assumptions in the development of DSM-III and DSM-III-R: an insider's perspective and a belated response to Sadler, Hugus and Agich's "on the values in recent American psychiatric classification." J Nerv Ment Dis. 2001;189:351–359.
11. Meehl PE. Bootstraps taxometrics. Solving the classification problem in psychopathology. Am Psychol. 1995;50:266–275.
12. Andreasen NC. Understanding schizophrenia: a silent spring? Am J Psychiatry. 1998;155:1657–1659.
13. Eaton WW, Romanoski A, Anthony JC, Nestadt G. Screening for psychosis in the general population with a self-report interview. J Nerv Ment Dis. 1991;179:689–693.
14. Janssen I, Hanssen M, Bak M, et al. Discrimination and delusional ideation. Br J Psychiatry. 2003;182:71–76.
15. Johns LC, Cannon M, Singleton N, et al. Prevalence and correlates of self-reported psychotic symptoms in the British population. Br J Psychiatry. 2004;185:298–305.

16. Kendler KS, Gallagher TJ, Abelson JM, Kessler RC. Lifetime prevalence, demographic risk factors, and diagnostic validity of nonaffective psychosis as assessed in a US community sample. The National Comorbidity Survey. Arch Gen Psychiatry. 1996;53:1022–1031.

17. King M, Nazroo J, Weich S, et al. Psychotic symptoms in the general population of England—a comparison of ethnic groups (The EMPIRIC study). Soc Psychiatry Psychiatr Epidemiol. 2005;40:375–381.

18. Olfson M, Lewis-Fernandez R, Weissman MM, et al. Psychotic symptoms in an urban general medicine practice. Am J Psychiatry. 2002;159:1412–1419.

19. Peters ER, Joseph SA, Garety PA. Measurement of delusional ideation in the normal population: introducing the PDI (Peters et al. Delusions Inventory). Schizophr Bull. 1999; 25:553–576.

20. Poulton R, Caspi A, Moffitt TE, Cannon M, Murray R, Harrington H. Children's self-reported psychotic symptoms and adult schizophreniform disorder: a 15-year longitudinal study. Arch Gen Psychiatry. 2000;57:1053–1058.

21. Tien AY. Distributions of hallucinations in the population. Soc Psychiatry Psychiatr Epidemiol. 1991;26:287–292.

22. van Os J, Hanssen M, Bijl RV, Ravelli A. Strauss (1969) revisited: a psychosis continuum in the general population? Schizophr Res. 2000;45:11–20.

23. van Os J, Hanssen M, Bijl RV, Vollebergh W. Prevalence of psychotic disorder and community level of psychotic symptoms: an urban-rural comparison. Arch Gen Psychiatry. 2001; 58:663–668.

24. Verdoux H, Maurice-Tison S, Gay B, van Os J, Salamon R, Bourgeois ML. A survey of delusional ideation in primary-care patients. Psychol Med. 1998;28:127–134.

25. Wiles NJ, Zammit S, Bebbington P, Singleton N, Meltzer H, Lewis G. Self-reported psychotic symptoms in the general population: results from the longitudinal study of the British National Psychiatric Morbidity Survey. Br J Psychiatry. 2006;188:519–526.

26. Bebbington P, Nayani T. The psychosis screening questionnaire. Int J Methods Psychiatr Res. 1995;5:11–19.

27. Chapman LJ, Chapman JP, Kwapil TR, Eckblad M, Zinser MC. Putatively psychosis-prone subjects 10 years later. J Abnorm Psychol. 1994;103:171–183.

28. McGlashan TH, Johannessen JO. Early detection and intervention with schizophrenia: rationale. Schizophr Bull. 1996;22:201–222.

29. Haertel EH. Continuous and discrete latent structure models for item response data. Psychometrika. 1990;55:477–494.

30. McCulloch CE, Lin H, Slate EH, Turnbell BW. Discovering subpopulation structure with latent class mixed models. Stat Med. 2002;21:417–429.

31. Lenzenweger MF. Consideration of the challenges, complications, and pitfalls of taxometric analysis. J Abnorm Psychol. 2004;113:10–23.

32. Murphy EA. One cause? Many causes? The argument from the bimodal distribution. J Chronic Dis. 1964;17:301–324.

33. Goldman-Rakic PS. More clues on "latent" schizophrenia point to developmental origins. Am J Psychiatry. 1995;152:1701–1703.

34. Kendell RE, Brockington IF. The identification of disease entities and the relationship between schizophrenia and affective psychosis. Br J Psychiatry. 1980;137:324–331.
35. Lindenmayer JP, Brown E, Baker RW, et al. An excitement subscale of the positive and negative syndrome scale. Schizophr Res. 2004;68:331–337.
36. van Os J, Gilvarry C, Bale R, et al. A comparison of the utility of dimensional and categorical representations of psychosis. UK700 Group. Psychol Med. 1999;29:595–606.
37. van Os J, Gilvarry C, Bale R, et al. Diagnostic value of the DSM and ICD categories of psychosis: an evidence-based approach. UK700 Group. Soc Psychiatry Psychiatr Epidemiol. 2000;35:305–311.
38. Ratakonda S, Gorman JM, Yale SA, Amador XF. Characterization of psychotic conditions. Use of the domains of psychopathology model. [see comment]. Arch Gen Psychiatry. 1998;55:75–81.
39. McGorry PD, Bell RC, Dudgeon PL, Jackson HJ. The dimensional structure of first episode psychosis: an exploratory factor analysis. Psychol Med. 1998;28:935–947.
40. Kendler KS, Karkowski LM, Prescott CA, Pedersen NL. Latent class analysis of temperance board registrations in Swedish male-male twin pairs born 1902 to 1949: searching for subtypes of alcoholism. Psychol Med. 1998;28:803–813.
41. Murray V, McKee I, Miller PM, et al. Dimensions and classes of psychosis in a population cohort: a four-class, four-dimension model of schizophrenia and affective psychoses. Psychol Med. 2005;35:499–510.
42. Andreasen NC, Olsen S. Negative v positive schizophrenia. Definition and validation. Arch Gen Psychiatry. 1982;39:789–794.
43. Carpenter WT, Heinrichs DW, Wagman AM. Deficit and nondeficit forms of schizophrenia: the concept. Am J Psychiatry. 1988;145:578–583.
44. Buchanan RW, Carpenter WT. Domains of psychopathology. An approach to the reduction of heterogeneity in schizophrenia. J Nerv Ment Dis. 1994;182:193–204.
45. Fenton WS, McGlashan TH. Antecedents, symptom progression and long term outcome of the deficit syndrome in schizophrenia. Am J Psychiatry. 1994;151:351–356.
46. Heckers S, Goff D, Schacter DL, et al. Functional imaging of memory retrieval in deficit vs nondeficit schizophrenia. Arch Gen Psychiatry. 1999;56:1117–1123.
47. Horan WP, Blanchard JJ. Neurocognitive, social and emotional dysfunction in deficit syndrome schizophrenia. Schizophr Res. 2003;65:125–137.
48. Kirkpatrick B, Buchanan RW. Anhedonia and the deficit syndrome of schizophrenia. Psychiatry Res. 1990;31:25–30.
49. Kirkpatrick B, Ross DE, Walsh D, Karkowski L, Kendler KS. Family characteristics of deficit and nondeficit schizophrenia in the Roscommon Family Study. Schizophr Res. 2000;45:57–64.
50. Kirkpatrick B, Tek C, Allardyce J, Morrison G, McCreadie RG. Summer birth and deficit schizophrenia in Dumfries and Galloway, southwestern Scotland. [see comment]. Am J Psychiatry. 2002;159:1382–1387.
51. Ross DE, Thaker GK, Buchanan RW, et al. Association of abnormal smooth pursuit eye movements with the deficit syndrome in schizophrenic patients. Am J Psychiatry. 1996;153:1158–1165.

52. Blanchard JJ, Horan WP, Collins LM. Examining the latent structure of negative symptoms: is there a distinct subtype of negative symptom schizophrenia? Schizophr Res. 2005;77:151–165.

53. Kessler RC. Epidemiological perspectives for the development of future diagnostic systems. Psychopathology. 2002;35:158–161.

54. Ruscio J, Ruscio AM. Clarifying boundary issues in psychopathology: the role of taxometrics in a comprehensive program of structural research. J Abnorm Psychol. 2004;113:24–38.

55. Grube BS, Bilder RM, Goldman RS. Meta-analysis of symptom factors in schizophrenia. Schizophr Res. 1998;31:113–120.

56. Serretti A, Rietschel M, Lattuada E, et al. Major psychoses symptomatology: factor analysis of 2241 psychotic subjects. Eur Arch Psychiatry Clin Neurosci. 2001;251:193–198.

57. Serretti A, Olgiati P. Dimensions of major psychoses: a confirmatory factor analysis of six competing models. Psychiatry Res. 2004;127:101–109.

58. McIntosh AM, Forrester A, Lawrie SM, et al. A factor model of the functional psychoses and the relationship of factors to clinical variables and brain morphology. Psychol Med. 2001;31:159–171.

59. Drake RJ, Dunn G, Tarrier N, Haddock G, Haley C, Lewis S. The evolution of symptoms in the early course of nonaffective psychosis. Schizophr Res. 2003;63:171–179.

60. Peralta V, Cuesta MJ, Giraldo C, Cardenas A, Gonzalez F. Classifying psychotic disorders: issues regarding categorical vs. dimensional approaches and time frame to assess symptoms. Eur Arch Psychiatry Clin Neurosci. 2002;252:12–18.

61. van Os J, Fahy TA, Jones P, et al. Psychopathological syndromes in the functional psychoses: associations with course and outcome. Psychol Med. 1996;26:161–176.

62. Rosenman S, Korten A, Medway J, Evans M. Dimensional vs. categorical diagnosis in psychosis. Acta Psychiatr Scand. 2003;107:378–384.

63. Gaebel W, Saß H. Psychopathologische Methoden und psychiatrische Forschung, in Objektivierende Psychopathologie in der biologisch–psychiatrischen Farschung. Edited by Saß H. Jena, Stuttgart, Germany: Gustav Fischer Verlag; 1996, pp 15–28.

64. Shallice T. From Neuropsychology to Mental Structure. Cambridge, England: Cambridge University Press; 1988.

2

BIOLOGICAL, LIFE COURSE, AND CROSS-CULTURAL STUDIES ALL POINT TOWARD THE VALUE OF DIMENSIONAL AND DEVELOPMENTAL RATINGS IN THE CLASSIFICATION OF PSYCHOSIS

Rina Dutta, MRCPsych
Talya Greene, Ph.D.
Jean Addington, Ph.D.
Kwame McKenzie, MRCPsych
Michael Phillips, M.D., M.P.H.
Robin M. Murray, M.D., D.Sc., FRCPsych, FMedSci

Reprinted with permission from Dutta R, Greene T, Addington J, McKenzie K, Phillips M, Murray RM. "Biological, Life Course, and Cross-Cultural Studies All Point Toward the Value of Dimensional and Developmental Ratings in the Classification of Psychosis." *Schizophrenia Bulletin* 2007; 33: 868–876.

The Recent History of the Classification of Psychoses in the West

For the categorical diagnosis of schizophrenia to be scientifically valid, it should define a syndrome with specific risk factors, psychopathology, treatment responses, and outcomes; clear symptom boundaries should separate it from other conditions such as the affective psychoses. That such a distinction could be made between "dementia praecox" and "manic depressive insanity" (schizophrenia and affective psychosis) has been fundamental to psychiatric classificatory systems since Kraepelin's original proposal of the dichotomy in the 19th century. This is despite the fact that in 1920 Kraepelin came to doubt his own approach and suggested replacing his defining principle with a dimensional-hierarchical model more appropriate to the heterogeneity of clinical presentations.[1] Furthermore, in spite of the theoretical distinction between schizophrenia and mood disorder with psychotic features, the practicalities of clinical life led to development of a less than satisfactory intermediate category—schizoaffective disorder.

ATTACKS ON THE CONCEPT OF SCHIZOPHRENIA

The 1960s saw a sustained attack on psychiatry from the so-called antipsychiatrists, including R. D. Lang and Thomas Szasz, curiously both psychiatrists, who argued that psychiatric diagnoses such as schizophrenia were arbitrary categories that did not correspond to clinical reality. Then in the 1990s, more academically sophisticated criticism came from British clinical psychologists such as Richard Bentall and Mary Boyle who argued that a symptom-based approach was less stigmatizing and more appropriate from a therapeutic point of view.[2,3] However, criticism did not just stem from outside orthodox psychiatry. Phenomenologists such as Brockington, biological researchers such as Crow, and epidemiologists such as van Os have led a growing chorus of dissent from within the ranks of psychiatrists.

THE HOPE PROMISED BY OPERATIONAL DEFINITIONS

From the late 1960s onward, a number of competing operational diagnostic systems were proposed in an attempt to improve the reliability of psychiatric diagnosis for research purposes. These included Feighner's, Taylor's, Schneider's, Langfeldt's, Spitzer's, Carpenter's, Astrachan's, two from Forrest and Hay, and the Present State Examination—CATEGO system. These operational definitions were generally shown to be internally reliable once psychiatrists were trained in their use. However, the various competing diagnostic systems were compared with respect to their reliability, concordance, and prediction of outcome[4,5] and found to show wide disparity. For example, the systems varied by as much as sevenfold in their rates of diagnosing schizophrenia.[6]

These criteria, which were primarily designed for research purposes, were followed by the incorporation of similar operational rules for clinicians in the third edition of the *Diagnostic and Statistical Manual of Mental Disorders* (DSM-III)[7] published in 1980. Like the Feighner criteria, the DSM-III definition of schizophrenia was narrow, requiring 6 months of illness before the diagnosis could be made.

In the Camberwell Register study conducted by Castle and colleagues,[8] the authors examined the proportion of patients with a first episode of nonaffective psychosis who met different criteria. Nearly two-thirds of the 486 cases met the Research Diagnostic Criteria for either "broad" or "narrow" schizophrenia; this is not surprising given that this is the most liberal system, with no age-at-onset stipulation and only a 2-week illness duration requirement. However, only 32.6% of 486 cases fulfilled the criteria for schizophrenia in DSM-III and 32.3% for definite schizophrenia by the Feighner criteria, remarkably similar proportions that reflect the fact that the DSM-III criteria were much influenced by the St. Louis school from which the Feighner criteria had emerged. Both the Feighner and DSM-III criteria had a high degree of predictive specificity, with one study showing no change in diagnosis over time using these criteria and an average of 6.5 years of follow-up.[9]

THE CONTINUING PROBLEM OF VALIDITY

With training, especially in the use of standardized interviews, DSM-III, like the other main competing systems, produced acceptable interrater reliability. However, reliability does not necessarily mean validity, and attempts to study validity as opposed to reliability were limited. Robins and Guze[10] suggested five criteria to establish the validity of psychiatric diagnoses and illustrated their applicability to schizophrenia, namely, clinical description, laboratory studies, delimitation from other disorders, follow-up studies, and family studies. Kendler[11] developed this approach by distinguishing between antecedent, concurrent, and predictive validators. However, although the intention in devising DSM-III was to use "research evidence relevant to various kinds of diagnostic validity"[7] including "the largest reliability study ever done,"[12] the committee chairman Robert Spitzer acknowledged that "the subjective judgment of the members of the task force…played a crucial role in the development of DSM-III, and differences of opinion could only rarely be resolved by appeal to objective data."[13]

In 1994, DSM-IV was published.[14] It shifted the emphasis on which psychotic symptoms were required for a diagnosis of schizophrenia, in that patients without either delusions or hallucinations could receive the diagnosis. In these cases, however, other characteristic psychotic symptoms were required, namely, gross disorganization of speech and/or behavior. The diagnostic importance of Schneiderian symptoms was also reemphasized, as hallucinations can satisfy a criterion if they involve one or more voices engaging in running commentary or ongoing conversation, and delusions can count if they are bizarre.[15]

However, to date, the DSM review process has not used external validators such as quantitative biological measurements or psychological testing to assist in the evaluation of diagnostic criteria or to judge whether changes are improving clinical validity. Furthermore, it did not prove better than the other systems, and ultimately it was the power and influence of the American Psychiatric Association rather than any innate scientific superiority of DSM-IV that determined that it became most widely accepted throughout the world.

An alternative to choosing between these definitions was to adopt a polydiagnostic approach, where several sets of criteria were applied to the same patients.[16,17] One tool was the Operation Criteria Checklist for psychotic illness.[18] This approach uses a suite of computer programs to generate diagnoses according to 13 different classification systems. It has been a useful adjunct to research methodology in light of the lack of a clear definition of the boundaries of schizophrenia and the wide variety of presentations. However, it is clearly impractical in everyday clinical practice.

SEARCHING FOR SUBTYPES

Another alternative to establishing clear-cut and defensible borders of schizophrenia was to suggest that it comprised several discrete subtypes and to use external criteria to try and validate these. The 1980s saw a number of attempts to account for diagnostic heterogeneity by probing for subtypes of schizophrenia, for example, positive, negative, and mixed schizophrenia[19]; familial and sporadic schizophrenia[20]; deficit and nondeficit schizophrenia[21]; and subtypes with some similarity to traditional hebephrenic and paranoid forms ("H" and "P" subtypes).[22] Murray and colleagues[23] later sought to discriminate developmental from adult onset forms. Support for their hypothesis came from latent class analyses, but there remained the problem of intermediate forms.[24,25] Furthermore, genetic and environmental risk factors were seen to operate across diagnostic categories.[26,27]

DSM-V:
A Parochial System for Use in Certain Parts of North America or an International System?

The reader will have noticed that the above discussion has been largely confined to proposals and papers emanating from Western countries, particularly the United States. The nosological paradigms developed to categorize different types of psychotic symptoms are embedded in specific professional cultures, but unfortunately, nosological discussions have rarely involved psychiatrists working in non-Western countries. This omission would be of little relevance to those preparing DSM-V if it was merely to be used in the United States. However, the power of the American Psychiatric Association and American psychiatry in general has resulted in DSM-IV becoming the de facto system adopted by researchers throughout large parts of the world, indeed in preference to the *International Classification of Diseases,* 10th Revision (ICD). Clearly, if DSM-V seeks to be an international system, then it must address issues outside those of the United States.

RESEARCH FROM NON-WESTERN COUNTRIES

Sadly, much of the research on psychotic conditions from developing countries—where the vast majority of individuals with psychotic conditions live—is unknown or dismissed as methodologically flawed by nosologists from developed countries. The substantial differences in the onset, course, and treatment response of psychotic symptoms between developed and less developed countries identified in the international pilot study on schizophrenia[28] have had little effect on the dominant theories of psychosis that have all been developed in Western countries and based on data from developed countries. Furthermore, studies that identify acute remitting psychosis[29] in developing countries have been largely disregarded by Western nosologists. It is often assumed that methodological problems produce the "aberrant" findings, and so no attempt is made to identify other, more complex, explanations.

Issues of Culture

Thus, little attention has been paid to the fact that experience and understanding of psychotic symptoms are embedded in a network of local meanings that vary from nation to nation, within different subcultural groups in a single nation, and over time (as communities undergo sociocultural changes). Culture influences an individual's perception of the world, the content of their thoughts, and therefore the form and quality of psychotic symptoms. It helps to determine the interpretation of symptoms and their subsequent social impact and guides both help seeking and the response to treatment. At a group level, culture can be considered important not only in defining and creating specific sources of stress and distress but also in providing specific modes of coping with distress and the social responses to distress and disability.[30,31]

A good example of subcultural differences in the attitudes and help-seeking behavior of patients with schizophrenia and their families comes from China, where there is a significant difference between patients from urban and rural areas.[32] In rural areas, mental illness is often associated with malevolent spirits, and therefore, many families seek help from witch doctors. One study found that 73.9% (*N*=286 of 387) of rural psychiatry outpatients admitted to previously consulting shamans,[33] whereas only 4.9% (N=21 of 426) of schizophrenia patients from an urban area in Beijing had done so.

A separate study suggested that while families of rural patients had a tendency to blame the illness on "external" factors such as spiritual forces, family members in urban areas were more likely to employ "internal" causal explanations. These included blaming the illness on pressure of studies, failure in love, or inability to adapt to a new competitive environment; less commonly used explanatory models involved physiological imbalances and psychological problems, such as personality quirks, excessive introversion, or nervousness.[34] There was also a higher perceived effect of stigma in urban areas. Urban patients with a young age of illness onset are less likely to receive government-sponsored employment and to find a spouse, and therefore, they are considered socially inferior.[35]

ISSUES CONCERNING ETHNICITY

An influential study carried out by the World Health Organization was interpreted by its authors and others to suggest that the incidence of schizophrenia was unvarying.[36] However, subsequent studies have demonstrated international, intranational, and cross-cultural differences in rates of psychotic illness.[37] Furthermore, differences in the rates of schizophrenia have also been demonstrated for minority ethnic groups within a country. Thus, increased rates have been reported for the diagnosis of schizophrenia in migrant groups in Demark, France, Sweden, The Netherlands, and the United Kingdom. A recent meta-analysis of published studies by Cantor-Graae and Selten[38] has demonstrated that different types of migrants have different risks of schizophrenia (Table 2–1).

The Curious Example of African Caribbeans in the United Kingdom

The group that has been most intensively studied is African Caribbeans in the United Kingdom, who show rates of psychosis several times that of the white British population (e.g., incidence rate ratios for schizophrenia 9.1 and manic psychosis 8.0 in a recent multicenter study[37]). Similarly high rates have not been reported for other immigrant groups, and the rates of psychosis in the Caribbean are not elevated. The increased risk seems not to be due to being an immigrant or being African Caribbean but being an immigrant from the Caribbean living in the United Kingdom.[39]

The evidence is that there is a significant impact of living or being born in the United Kingdom, which puts those African Caribbeans already at genetic risk of developing schizophrenia at an even greater risk.[40] Genetic vulnerability and the social/environmental context appear to be acting together in this cultural group to markedly increase rates.

Are the higher rates of psychosis in the African Caribbean UK population due to real increased rates of schizophrenia or are they due to misdiagnosis? In one study, a Jamaican psychiatrist was asked to make diagnoses on African Caribbean inpatients at

TABLE 2–1.   Based on published meta-analyses of population-based studies examining the association between migration and risk of schizophrenia

Migrant group	Relative risk	95% CI
First-generation migrants	2.7	2.3–3.2
Second-generation migrants	4.5	1.5–13.1
Migrants with "black" skin color	4.8	3.7–6.2
Migrants with "white" skin color	2.3	1.7–3.1

a London teaching hospital. While the UK doctors diagnosed schizophrenia in 52% of patients and the Jamaican psychiatrist diagnosed schizophrenia in 55% of patients, the two only agreed on the diagnosis of schizophrenia in 55% of patients.[41] The results were no different whether ICD or DSM was used. This suggests problems in the reliability of diagnosing schizophrenia but not of racial bias in application of diagnosis.[42]

The difficulty in categorizing psychiatric illness is further underlined by differences in the course of schizophrenia between the African Caribbean community and native whites in the United Kingdom. African Caribbeans are approximately 40% less likely to suffer from a continuous illness than British whites,[43] and it is suggested that they are less likely to have a history of obstetric complications or neurological illness premorbidly.[44] It has been hypothesized that the good symptomatic prognosis reflects increased rates of illness in less neurologically and genetically vulnerable people who have had relatively normal early development but have been exposed to social stressors that have promoted psychosis. One possible contributing factor is racial discrimination. Studies show that the darker the skin color, the more racism an individual is subject to regardless of mental illness.[45] One longitudinal study has demonstrated that those who experience discrimination are at an increased risk of developing delusional ideation.[46] The lesson of these studies is that there may be a different balance of causes of psychosis, a different spectrum of symptoms, and a different outcome of psychosis in different populations.

Findings From Recent Biological Studies
PHARMACOLOGY

Evidence that schizophrenia and bipolar disorder are not as dissimilar as the neo-Kraepelinian view suggests comes from studies showing that antipsychotics are effective in both conditions, thus implicating dopamine dysregulation as a key common mechanism in their etiology.[47] For years, the responsiveness of bipolar disorder to lithium and other mood stabilizers was taken as a feature classically distinguishing it from schizophrenia. Recently, however, significant reduction in the severity of symptoms was observed in patients with an acute exacerbation of schizophrenia in whom divalproex was added in to olanzapine or risperidone treatment.[48] This builds upon earlier work by Brockington[49] that showed that lithium and chlorpromazine were equally effective in schizoaffective patients and detracts from a notion that there are distinct psychotic disorders with unique treatment pathways.

GENETICS

Schizophrenia and bipolar disorder occur together in the same families more frequently than chance. Furthermore, in a twin study using blinded diagnostic assessments and relaxing the normal hierarchical approach whereby schizophrenia trumps all other diagnoses, Cardno et al.[50] showed that if one member of a monozygotic twin pair has schizophrenia, there is about an 8% chance of the co-twin being diagnosed with schizoaffective disorder and an 8% chance of mania being diagnosed instead. Furthermore, as discussed elsewhere in this volume, recent molecular genetic studies, although as yet preliminary, suggest overlap between risk genes for schizophrenia and bipolar disorder.[51]

NEUROIMAGING

Brain morphometry studies have shown that schizophrenia is associated with distributed gray matter deficits particularly in the frontotemporal neocortex, medial temporal lobe, insula, thalamus, and cerebellum, whereas patients with bipolar disorder have no significant areas of gray matter abnormality. However, both disorders show anatomically coincident white matter abnormalities in regions normally occupied by major longitudinal and interhemispheric tracts.[52]

A Developmental Perspective

Thus, pharmacological, genetic, and neuroimaging studies suggest both similarities and differences between schizophrenia and bipolar disorder. Some understanding of the basis of these comes from adopting a life course perspective on the illnesses. Numerous studies have shown that preschizophrenic children are characterized by impairments in cognitive and neuromotor development. This was demonstrated very clearly in the Dunedin study, which was also the first to demonstrate that these [impairments] are not a feature of those who later develop bipolar disorder.[53]

Confirmation that bipolar patients do not have general neurocognitive impairment is provided by the Israeli Draft Board Registry study,[54] which showed that 68 individuals hospitalized with bipolar disorder did not differ from their healthy matched counterparts on any test of intellectual, language, or behavioral functioning conducted routinely when they were adolescents. A more recent co-

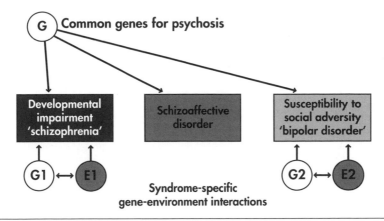

FIGURE 2–1. Gene-environment interactions to explain the overlap and distinctions between schizophrenia and bipolar disorder (after Cardno et al.[50] and Murray et al.[58]).

hort study using national registers to follow all Swedish children who completed compulsory education showed that no students with excellent school performance developed schizophrenia or schizoaffective disorder. By contrast, achieving outstanding grades in certain school subjects was a significant predictor of later bipolar disorder.[55]

Further evidence that schizophrenia and bipolar disorders are at least partially distinct in etiology comes from studying complications of pregnancy and delivery. Obstetric events have been described as being more frequent in schizophrenia.[56,57] Perinatal hypoxia arising from birth complications is particularly known to affect growth of the amygdala and hippocampus, which are often reported to be smaller in schizophrenia and not in bipolar disorder.[58] There is no substantive evidence that obstetric complications increase the risk of bipolar disorder.[59] Moreover, fetal growth indicators such as birth weight, birth length, and gestational age have also not been identified as risk factors for bipolar disorder.[60]

The similarities and differences between schizophrenia and bipolar disorder begin to suggest a model (Figure 2–1) in which given a shared background of genetic predisposition to psychosis, additional specific genetic or early environmental insults interact to impair neurodevelopment, leaving individuals vulnerable to schizophrenia. By contrast, in bipolar disorder, developmental impairment is absent but syndrome-specific genes and environmental interactions may render individuals susceptible to social adversity.

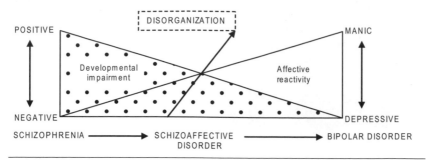

FIGURE 2–2. Schema incorporating five dimensions (after van Os et al.[63]) and explaining the "spectrum" of syndromes from schizophrenia through to bipolar disorder.

A Dimensional Perspective

Traditionally, first-rank symptoms are given particular emphasis for making a diagnosis of schizophrenia rather than bipolar disorder. However, although Cardno and colleagues[61] showed that a syndrome characterized by the presence of one or more first-rank symptoms has considerable heritability (71%, 95% confidence interval [CI] 57–82, compatible with a genetic contribution to variance in liability), it remains somewhat lower than that for schizophrenia as defined by established classifications, including DSM criteria.

An alternative to considering syndrome-based approaches to psychopathology is to use identified groups of correlated symptoms (symptom dimensions) in patient populations that comprise a range of diagnostic groups[62] (shown schematically in Figure 2–2). Different research teams have extracted usually four or five different factors or dimensions (e.g., depressive, manic, positive, negative, and disorganization symptoms), and broadly these have been remarkably consistent between studies of different patient cohorts.

Recently, it has been shown that using such symptom dimensions explains more about disease characteristics (such as premorbid impairment, the existence of stressors before disease onset, poor remissions or no recovery between episodes and exacerbations, response to neuroleptics, and deterioration) than diagnoses alone and thus adds substantial information to diagnostic categories.[64]

PSYCHOSIS AS A DIMENSION REACHING INTO THE GENERAL POPULATION

Various groups have in recent years pointed out that minor psychotic symptoms occur in the general population[65–67] and that psychosis is best conceived as a di-

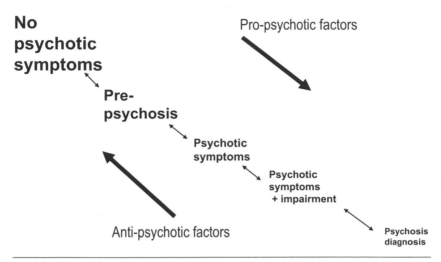

FIGURE 2–3.　A risk pathway to the diagnosis of psychosis.

mension like hypertension rather than a distinct category. (Refer to the review of Allardyce et al.[68] for further discussion of dimensional representations of psychotic illness.) Further evidence also comes from studies of those at ultra high risk of developing psychosis.

There is ample evidence that psychosis is "brewing" long before its manifestation as a diagnosable illness[69] and that identifiable signs and symptoms preceding the development of frank psychotic symptoms are evident.[70] DSM-IV criteria for schizophrenia include this "prodromal phase" as a construct, but it describes a retrospective concept because it cannot be defined until there is an established psychotic illness. DSM-III identified nine symptoms considered to be "prodromal" for schizophrenia and included them as diagnostic contributors. However, in a study by the Melbourne group based on retrospective conceptualization, these nine symptoms were found to have specificities between 0.58 and 0.88 and positive predictive values between 0.36 and 0.48 but were not pathognomic of schizophrenic psychosis.[71]

Indeed, in one study, Yung and colleagues[72] reported that for those ultra high-risk individuals who subsequently developed psychosis, diagnoses ranged from schizophrenia, through schizoaffective disorder, brief psychotic disorder, bipolar disorder to major depression. Using current "ultra high-risk" criteria, it appears as if early signs and symptoms are predictive of conversion to a spectrum of psychotic disorders but not of the exact nature of the psychosis that will develop.

It seems that the final diagnosis of a psychotic illness is merely the endpoint of a risk pathway that in itself is a slippery slope but not inevitable trajectory into psychosis (Figure 2–3); this view is very compatible with the dimensional view of psy-

chosis already discussed. In many cases, the pathway includes the development of
prepsychotic symptoms, the development of frank but infrequent psychotic symptoms, the development of persistent psychotic symptoms, and finally social impairment due to these psychotic symptoms. Moving up or down the pathway
depends on a balance between propsychotic factors such as individual biological
vulnerability, the use of cannabis, and the social environment and antipsychotic
factors such as individual resilience.

A Scheme Incorporating Developmental and Dimensional Ratings Offers a Possible Way Forward

There is great dissatisfaction with the DSM-IV concept of schizophrenia within
North America, considerably more in Europe, and psychiatrists from the developing world regard it as largely ignoring the issues of three-quarters of the globe. Difficulties in diagnosing mental illness among ethnic minority groups highlight the
need for a universal classification system that can be effectively applied. However,
the difference in rates of psychotic illness between countries and among different
ethnic groups within a country also suggest that viewing culture and ethnicity as
confounding variables in the conceptualization of mental illness is misguided.
Rather, culture and ethnicity ought to be seen as fundamental elements driving its
expression and interpretation.

By considering psychotic disorders from a life course perspective, including genetic factors, neurodevelopmental distinctions, symptomatology, structural neuroimaging, treatment strategies, and groups at ultra high risk of psychosis, we can
see that a scheme that takes into consideration both developmental and dimensional characteristics as discussed above appears a possible way forward. For example, those at ultra high risk of psychosis would be rated at points on dimensions
compatible with the extent and severity of their psychotic symptoms and affective
symptoms. Whether or not they showed evidence of developmental impairment
would help to predict the clinical picture of a full-blown psychosis if and when it
developed. Again, as applied to African Caribbeans with psychosis in the United
Kingdom, such a model would suggest that this population is more vulnerable to
a largely nondevelopmental illness in which social etiological factors are particularly important and which may present with a mixture of schizophrenic and manic
symptoms.

However, whether diagnoses are based on symptom dimensions or diagnostic
categories, the instruments for rating symptoms have typically been developed by
selecting a subset of useful items from a large preliminary pool of items based on
the results of a series of studies involving subjects in Western countries. If the en-

tire process was repeated in a non-Western country, it would almost inevitably result in a very different instrument with different items and a different factor structure. For example, studies in China on symptom scales in schizophrenia[73] have clearly demonstrated that translated and back-translated instruments can often achieve satisfactory test-retest reliability, but substantial revision is needed in order to achieve internal consistency and validity.

Another problem seen in the use of Western diagnostic instruments in developing countries is the assumption that a single probe is sufficient to elicit a particular symptom; this is particularly problematic in fully structured diagnostic instruments that do not allow the interviewer to revise the question based on the educational and cultural background of the respondent. This single-probe method may work in developed countries where the experience and expression of psychological symptoms has been "homogenized" by frequent media exposure and other social forces; but for example in China, the huge sociocultural differences between urban and rural residents make it necessary to employ multiple probes to capture the different methods of experiencing and describing specific psychological symptoms.[74]

Thus, if the DSM-V system of classifying psychosis is to be relevant to patients in the developing world, then instruments aimed at either making diagnoses or rating symptoms have to be subject to much more sophisticated field studies in non-Western countries than hitherto.

Proposal of a Hybrid System

It is clear that the categories of psychosis as used currently in DSM-IV are not valid in a strictly scientific sense. Their replacement by a developmental and dimensional approach as outlined above has much to recommend it for DSM-V. However, the current system does have some utility in terms of the information about etiology, course of illness, outcome, and treatment response that the different diagnoses convey.[75] Abandoning it would be a very dramatic shift, and although we believe it would be an advance, some information of benefit to patients and clinicians would be lost.

We consider that at present the best option is to implement a hybrid of a categorical-dimensional approach in DSM-V. This would introduce the benefit of increased explanatory power of clinical characteristics without completely dismissing the traditional paradigm of the Kraepelinian dichotomy. Similarly, including a rating of developmental impairment would aid understanding of the longitudinal course of illness evolution, rather than considering a diagnosis as a cross-sectional perspective based only on the current clinical picture. Anything more radical is likely to be premature, with the expectation of further advances in genetic, neurobiological, environmental, and psychosocial research in the coming decade.

In parallel with research in individual disciplines, what is needed is a concerted multicenter effort to look back at existing epidemiologically based first-onset psychosis cohorts to investigate how external summary variables, including measures of cognition, social variables, and need for care, as well as symptom dimensions, familial liability scores, and basic structural magnetic resonance imaging data may sharpen the discriminative potential of the DSM classification of psychotic disorders. This should include cohort data from both developing and developed countries.

From our exploration of cultural issues, we suggest that standardized qualitative and quantitative methods need to be developed that can be employed in a wide range of different communities to conduct culturally sensitive assessments of psychotic symptoms. Only then will it be possible for the nosologist to attempt to identify universal "gold standard" criteria (preferably with unique biological and psychosocial markers) for a discrete set of psychotic diagnoses.

References

1. Kraepelin E. The manifestations of insanity [Die Erscheinungsformen des Irreseins]. Hist Psychiatry. 1992;3:509–529.
2. Bentall RP. Reconstructing Schizophrenia. London: Routledge; 1990.
3. Boyle M. Schizophrenia—A Scientific Delusion? London: Routledge; 1990.
4. Brockington IF, Kendell RE, Leff JP. Definitions of schizophrenia: concordance and prediction of outcome. Psychol Med. 1978;8:387–398.
5. Kendell RE, Brockington IF, Leff JP. Prognostic implications of six alternative definitions of schizophrenia. Arch Gen Psychiatry. 1979;36:25–31.
6. Endicott J. Diagnostic criteria for schizophrenia: reliabilities and agreement between systems. Arch Gen Psychiatry. 1982;39:884–889.
7. American Psychiatric Association. Diagnostic and Statistical Manual of Mental Disorders. 3rd ed. Washington, DC: American Psychiatric Association; 1980.
8. Castle DJ, Wessely S, van Os J, Murray RM. Diagnostic issues and admission policies. In: Psychosis in the Inner City: The Camberwell First Episode Study. London: Maudsley Monograph; 1998:19–25.
9. Helzer JE, Brockington IF, Kendell RE. Predictive validity of DSM-III and Feighner definitions of schizophrenia: a comparison with research diagnostic criteria and CATEGO. Arch Gen Psychiatry. 1981;38:791–797.
10. Robins E, Guze SB. Establishment of diagnostic validity in psychiatric illness: its application to schizophrenia. Am J Psychiatry. 1970;126:983–987.
11. Kendler KS. The nosologic validity of paranoia (simple delusional disorder): a review. Arch Gen Psychiatry. 1980;37:699–706.
12. Spitzer RL, Williams JB, Skodol AE. DSM-III: the major achievements and an overview. Am J Psychiatry. 1980;137:151–164.
13. Spitzer RL. DSM-III and the politics-science dichotomy syndrome: a response to Thomas E. Schacht's "DSM-III and the politics of truth." Am Psychol. 1985;40:522–526.

14. American Psychiatric Association. Diagnostic and Statistical Manual of Mental Disorders. 4th ed. Washington, DC: American Psychiatric Association; 1994.

15. Tsuang MT, Stone WS, Faraone SV. Toward reformulating the diagnosis of schizophrenia. Am J Psychiatry. 2000;157:1041–1050.

16. Berner P, Katschnig H, Lenz G. Poly-diagnostic approach: a method to clarify incongruences among the classification of the functional psychoses. Psychiatr J Univ Ott. 1982;7:244–248.

17. Jansson LB, Parnas J. Competing definitions of schizophrenia: what can be learned from polydiagnostic studies? Schizophr Bull. December 8, 2006; doi:10.1093/schbul/sbl065.

18. Farmer AE, Wessely S, Castle D, McGuffin P. Methodological issues in using a polydiagnostic approach to define psychotic illness. Br J Psychiatry. 1992;161:824–830.

19. Andreasen NC, Olsen S. Negative v positive schizophrenia. Definition and validation. Arch Gen Psychiatry. 1982;39:789–794.

20. Murray RM, Lewis SW, Reveley AM. Towards an aetiological classification of schizophrenia. Lancet. 1985;1:1023–1026.

21. Carpenter WT Jr, Buchanan RW, Kirkpatrick B, Tamminga C, Wood F. Strong inference, theory testing, and the neuroanatomy of schizophrenia. Arch Gen Psychiatry. 1993;50:825–831.

22. Farmer AE, McGuffin P, Gottesman II. Searching for the split in schizophrenia: a twin study perspective. Psychiatry Res. 1984;13:109–118.

23. Murray RM, O'Callaghan E, Castle DJ, Lewis SW. A neurodevelopmental approach to the classification of schizophrenia. Schizophr Bull. 1992;18:319–332.

24. Castle DJ, Sham PC, Wessely S, Murray RM. The subtyping of schizophrenia in men and women: a latent class analysis. Psychol Med. 1994;24:41–51.

25. Sham PC, Castle DJ, Wessely S, Farmer AE, Murray RM. Further exploration of a latent class typology of schizophrenia. Schizophr Res. 1996;20:105–115.

26. Done DJ, Crow TJ, Johnstone EC, Sacker A. Childhood antecedents of schizophrenia and affective illness: social adjustment at ages 7 and 11. BMJ. 1994;309:699–703.

27. van Os J, Jones P, Lewis G, Wadsworth M, Murray R. Developmental precursors of affective illness in a general population birth cohort. Arch Gen Psychiatry. 1997;54:625–631.

28. Sartorius N, Gulbinat W, Harrison G, Laska E, Siegel C. Long term follow-up of schizophrenia in 16 countries. A description of the International Study of Schizophrenia conducted by the World Health Organization. Soc Psychiatry Psychiatr Epidemiol. 1996;31:249–258.

29. Susser E, Wanderling J. Epidemiology of nonaffective acute remitting psychosis vs schizophrenia. Sex and sociocultural setting. Arch Gen Psychiatry. 1994;51:294–301.

30. Alarcon RD, Westermeyer J, Foulks EF, Ruiz P. Clinical relevance of contemporary cultural psychiatry. J Nerv Ment Dis. 1999;187:465–471.

31. Kirmayer LJ, Young A. Culture and context in the evolutionary concept of mental disorder. J Abnorm Psychol. 1999;108:446–452.

32. Phillips MR. The transformation of China's mental health services. China J. 1998;39:1–36.

33. Li SX, Phillips MR. Witch doctors and mental illness in mainland China: a preliminary study. Am J Psychiatry. 1990;147:221–224.
34. Phillips MR, Li Y, Stroup TS, Xin L. Causes of schizophrenia reported by patients' family members in China. Br J Psychiatry. 2000;177:20–25.
35. Phillips MR, Pearson V, Li F, Xu M, Yang L. Stigma and expressed emotion: a study of people with schizophrenia and their family members in China. Br J Psychiatry. 2002;181:488–493.
36. Jablensky A, Sartorius N, Ernberg G, et al. Schizophrenia: manifestations, incidence and course in different cultures. A World Health Organization ten-country study. Psychol Med Monogr Suppl. 1992;20:1–97.
37. Fearon P, Kirkbride JB, Morgan C, et al. Incidence of schizophrenia and other psychoses in ethnic minority groups: results from the MRC AESOP study. Psychol Med. 2006;1–10.
38. Cantor-Graae E, Selten JP. Schizophrenia and migration: a meta-analysis and review. Am J Psychiatry. 2005;162:12–24.
39. Fearon P, Morgan C. Environmental factors in schizophrenia: the role of migrant studies. Schizophr Bull. 2006;32:405–408.
40. Hutchinson G, Takei N, Fahy TA, et al. Morbid risk of schizophrenia in first-degree relatives of white and African-Caribbean patients with psychosis. Br J Psychiatry. 1996;169:776–780.
41. Hickling FW, McKenzie K, Mullen R, Murray R. A Jamaican psychiatrist evaluates diagnoses at a London psychiatric hospital. Br J Psychiatry. 1999;175:283–285.
42. Sharpley M, Hutchinson G, McKenzie K, Murray RM. Understanding the excess of psychosis among the African-Caribbean population in England. Review of current hypotheses. Br J Psychiatry Suppl. 2001;40:s60–s68.
43. McKenzie K, Samele C, van Horn E, Tattan T, van Os J, Murray R. Comparison of the outcome and treatment of psychosis in people of Caribbean origin living in the UK and British Whites: report from the UK700 trial. Br J Psychiatry. 2001;178:160–165.
44. McKenzie K, Jones P, Lewis S, et al. Lower prevalence of pre-morbid neurological illness in African-Caribbean than White psychotic patients in England. Psychol Med. 2002;32:1285–1291.
45. Klonoff EA, Landrine H. Is skin color a marker for racial discrimination? Explaining the skin color-hypertension relationship. J Behav Med. 2000;23:329–338.
46. Janssen I, Hanssen M, Bak M, et al. Discrimination and delusional ideation. Br J Psychiatry. 2003;182:71–76.
47. Post RM. Comparative pharmacology of bipolar disorder and schizophrenia. Schizophr Res. 1999;39:153–158.
48. Casey DE, Daniel DG, Wassef AA, Tracy KA, Wozniak P, Sommerville KW. Effect of divalproex combined with olanzapine or risperidone in patients with an acute exacerbation of schizophrenia. Neuropsychopharmacology. 2003;28:182–192.
49. Brockington IF, Kendell RE, Kellett JM, Curry SH, Wainwright S. Trials of lithium, chlorpromazine and amitriptyline in schizoaffective patients. Br J Psychiatry. 1978;133:162–168.
50. Cardno AG, Rijsdijk FV, Sham PC, Murray RM, McGuffin P. A twin study of genetic relationships between psychotic symptoms. Am J Psychiatry. 2002;159:539–545.

51. Craddock N, O'Donovan MC, Owen MJ. Genes for schizophrenia and bipolar disorder? Implications for psychiatric nosology. Schizophr Bull. 2006;32:9–16.

52. McDonald C, Bullmore E, Sham P, et al. Regional volume deviations of brain structure in schizophrenia and psychotic bipolar disorder: computational morphometry study. Br J Psychiatry. 2005;186:369–377.

53. Cannon M, Caspi A, Moffitt TE, et al. Evidence for early childhood, pan-developmental impairment specific to schizophreniform disorder: results from a longitudinal birth cohort. Arch Gen Psychiatry. 2002;59:449–456.

54. Reichenberg A, Weiser M, Rabinowitz J, et al. A population-based cohort study of premorbid intellectual, language, and behavioral functioning in patients with schizophrenia, schizoaffective disorder, and nonpsychotic bipolar disorder. Am J Psychiatry. 2002;159:2027–2035.

55. Maccabe J, Lambe M, Cnattingius S, et al. Academic achievement at age 16 has contrasting effects on risk of later bipolar disorder and schizophrenia. Schizophr Res. 2006;81(suppl):4–5.

56. Geddes JR, Verdoux H, Takei N, et al. Schizophrenia and complications of pregnancy and labor: an individual patient data meta-analysis. Schizophr Bull. 1999;25:413–423.

57. Cannon M, Jones PB, Murray RM. Obstetric complications and schizophrenia: historical and meta-analytic review. Am J Psychiatry. 2002;159:1080–1092.

58. Murray RM, Sham P, Zanelli J, Cannon M, McDonald C. A developmental model for similarities and dissimilarities between schizophrenia and bipolar disorder. Schizophr Res. 2004;71:405–416.

59. Scott J, McNeill Y, Cavanagh J, Cannon M, Murray R. Exposure to obstetric complications and subsequent development of bipolar disorder: systematic review. Br J Psychiatry. 2006;189:3–11.

60. Ogendahl BK, Agerbo E, Byrne M, Licht RW, Eaton WW, Mortensen PB. Indicators of fetal growth and bipolar disorder: a Danish national register-based study. Psychol Med. 2006;36:1219–1224.

61. Cardno AG, Sham PC, Farmer AE, Murray RM, McGuffin P. Heritability of Schneider's first-rank symptoms. Br J Psychiatry. 2002;180:35–38.

62. van Os J, Gilvarry C, Bale R, et al. A comparison of the utility of dimensional and categorical representations of psychosis. UK700 Group. Psychol Med. 1999;29:595–606.

63. van Os J, Gilvarry C, Bale R, et al. Diagnostic value of the DSM and ICD categories of psychosis: an evidence-based approach. UK700 Group. Soc Psychiatry Psychiatr Epidemiol. 2000;35:305–311.

64. Dikeos DG, Wickham H, McDonald C, et al. Distribution of symptom dimensions across Kraepelinian divisions. Br J Psychiatry. 2006;189:346–353.

65. van Os J, Hanssen M, Bijl RV, Ravelli A. Strauss (1969) revisited: a psychosis continuum in the general population? Schizophr Res. 2000;45:11–20.

66. Johns LC, Cannon M, Singleton N, et al. Prevalence and correlates of self-reported psychotic symptoms in the British population. Br J Psychiatry. 2004;185:298–305.

67. Wiles NJ, Zammit S, Bebbington P, Singleton N, Meltzer H, Lewis G. Self-reported psychotic symptoms in the general population: results from the longitudinal study of the British National Psychiatric Morbidity Survey. Br J Psychiatry. 2006;188:519–526.

68. Allardyce J, Gaebel W, Zielasek J, van Os J. Deconstructing Psychosis Conference February 2006: The Validity of Schizophrenia and Alternative Approaches to the Classification of Psychosis. Schizophr Bull. June 4, 2007; doi:10.1093/schbul/sbm051.

69. Poulton R, Caspi A, Moffitt TE, Cannon M, Murray R, Harrington H. Children's self-reported psychotic symptoms and adult schizophreniform disorder: a 15-year longitudinal study. Arch Gen Psychiatry. 2000;57:1053–1058.

70. McGlashan TH, Zipursky RB, Perkins D, et al. The PRIME North America randomized double-blind clinical trial of olanzapine versus placebo in patients at risk of being prodromally symptomatic for psychosis. I. Study rationale and design. Schizophr Res. 2003;61:7–18.

71. Jackson HJ, McGorry PD, Dudgeon P. Prodromal symptoms of schizophrenia in first-episode psychosis: prevalence and specificity. Compr Psychiatry. 1995;36:241–250.

72. Yung AR, Phillips LJ, Yuen HP, et al. Psychosis prediction: 12-month follow up of a high-risk ("prodromal") group. Schizophr Res. 2003;60:21–32.

73. Phillips MR, Xiong W, Wang RW, Gao YH, Wang XQ, Zhang NP. Reliability and validity of the Chinese versions of the Scales for Assessment of Positive and Negative Symptoms. Acta Psychiatr Scand. 1991;84:364–370.

74. Phillips MR, Shen QJ, Liu XH, et al. Assessing depressive symptoms in persons who die of suicide in mainland China. J Affect Disord. 2007;98:73–82.

75. Kendell R, Jablensky A. Distinguishing between the validity and utility of psychiatric diagnoses. Am J Psychiatry. 2003;160:4–12.

3

CURRENT ISSUES IN THE CLASSIFICATION OF PSYCHOTIC MAJOR DEPRESSION

Jennifer Keller, Ph.D.
Alan F. Schatzberg, M.D.
Mario Maj, M.D., Ph.D.

Depression is one of the most common mental disorders worldwide, with a current prevalence estimated between 2.1% and 7.6%.[1–4] A number of depressive subtypes have been identified, and there has been much debate about how to most accurately describe them. The current state of designating major depression with psychotic features (psychotic major depression, PMD) under the severity dimension is less than optimal, leading to two pressing issues. First, should PMD be classified as a separate subtype of major depression? Second, what should or could be done to improve the current severity dimension classification?

The prevalence of psychotic depression suggests that it is worth examining a reclassification. A recent study[5,6] reported that in the general population in five

Reprinted with permission from Keller J, Schatzberg AF, Maj M. "Current Issues in the Classification of Psychotic Major Depression." *Schizophrenia Bulletin* 2007; 33: 877–885. This article was supported in part by grants from the Pritzker Foundation and National Institutes of Health MH50604 to Alan Schatzberg.

European countries, 2.4% of those surveyed met criteria for unipolar major depression, of whom nearly 19% also had psychotic features. Thus, this study reported a prevalence of 0.4% of major depression with psychotic features. The percentage of major depressives with psychotic features is consistent with estimates of 15% of major depressives reporting a lifetime history of psychosis in the United States.[7]

There has been significant progress made in the last 10 years in our knowledge and understanding of PMD. There are considerable data to suggest that PMD and nonpsychotic major depression (NPMD) are separate syndromes, with different biological features, treatment response, and clinical course.[8,9] However, there are those who argue that the data are not uniformly consistent and that the discriminators may not be sensitive or specific enough to warrant a totally separate designation. A complete discussion of this debate is beyond the scope of this chapter, and the readers are referred to the last major review on this topic.[9] Even if one does not designate the disorder as a separate syndrome, the current severity dimension classification schemata have many problems and need to be revised. In this chapter, we first update the status of key potential characteristics and then discuss new dimensional solutions to classifying major depression.

Clinical Symptoms

Research suggests that specific symptoms appear to be more severe in PMD patients. For example, Rothschild et al.[10] reported that while PMD patients had higher depression scores than NPMD, this was primarily due to elevations on the retardation and cognitive disturbance items in PMD patients. Researchers have consistently reported more frequent and severe psychomotor difficulties (either agitation or retardation)[11,12] and increased feelings of guilt[12–14] in PMD.

In a recent article, Keller et al.[15] reported that PMD and NPMD patients, roughly matched for endogenous symptoms, were readily distinguished by ratings of the Positive Symptom Subscale (PSS) on the Brief Psychiatric Rating Scale[16] (BPRS), particularly the Unusual Thought Content (UTC) item. Very mild UTC endorsement, which indicates symptoms that fall short of being fully delusional, was an indicator of PMD. Moreover, the results suggested that any elevation, even very mild, on the PSS of the BPRS (i.e., conceptual disorganization, suspiciousness, hallucinations, and UTC) was even better at differentiating PMD from NMPD patients. Sensitivity and specificity for this scale were 84% and 99%, respectively. Beyond delusions and hallucinations, Parker and colleagues[14] found that PMDs were distinct from NPMD melancholic patients on psychomotor disturbance, depressive content, diurnal variation, and constipation. Even when researchers have matched patients for total depression scores, PMD patients demonstrated higher scores on psychomotor disturbances.[13]

A number of other symptoms have been reported to be greater in PMDs as compared with NPMDs, including depressed mood, paranoia, hypochondriasis, and anxiety. However, the empirical support for these is less robust and less consistent than are data supporting higher levels of UTC, psychomotor disturbances, and increased guilt. Thus, it appears that, although PMDs often have higher depression scores, this is likely due to specific, rather than a global, symptom elevation.

Clinical Course

The course of the depressive episodes has been found to be different in those who also exhibit psychotic features. Indeed, PMD patients often have longer duration of episodes [17,18] and a greater likelihood of recurrence of depression.[12,19] Moreover, patients with an index episode of psychotic depression tend to have previous episodes with psychosis.[9,11,20] Most of the studies, however, have been retrospective. In a recent prospective study, Maj and colleagues[18] found that the time to syndromal recovery from index episode was longer for PMDs than for nonpsychotic depressed patients.

There is some suggestion that PMDs have a higher morbidity as well as a higher suicide rate, although the latter is controversial.[21,22] In their 10-year follow-up study of 452 patients with an index episode of major depression, Maj et al.[18] found that the presence of delusions (but not of sustained preoccupations) in that episode was associated with a higher depressive morbidity during the prospective observation period, but not with a worse psychopathological and psychosocial outcome at the 10-year follow-up interview. This may indicate that the prognostic significance of delusions in major depression tends to become weaker over the long term, in line with the observation by Coryell and Tsuang.[23] Vythilingam et al.[22] also found that psychotic depression was associated with a twofold increase in mortality compared with depression without psychotic features. These findings held true after controlling for age and additional medical illness and were not due to elevated suicide rates. Overall, patients with psychotic depression tend to have longer duration of episodes, greater recurrence, and greater morbidity than those with nonpsychotic depression.

Familial History

Relatively little is known about familial history of unipolar major depression with psychotic features. Although we know that other specific psychiatric illnesses such as bipolar disorder and schizophrenia tend to be familial,[24,25] there are limited data on psychotic depression. A few early studies have reported that patients with PMD had an increased risk of family prevalence of unipolar major depression[26,27] and bipolar I disorder.[26] Others have found that family history of unipolar depression was similar between PMD and NPMD patients.[23]

A relationship between PMD and bipolar disorder has been repeatedly suggested on the basis of family history.[28] In their recent prospective follow-up study of 452 patients with an index episode of major depression, Maj et al.[18] found that patients with delusions in their index episode were significantly more likely to have a family history of bipolar I disorder than those without either delusions or sustained preoccupations. Moreover, 10.1% of patients with delusions in their index episode had a manic or hypomanic episode during the 10-year follow-up, compared with 3.2% of patients who had sustained preoccupations but not delusions in their index episode, and 5.0% of those without either delusions or sustained preoccupations. The switch to bipolarity was significantly associated with an earlier first psychiatric contact and a family history of bipolar I disorder but not with the presence of delusions in the index episode. Early-onset psychotic depression has been associated with a likely bipolar course in other studies.[29,30] More systematic gathering of family data for unipolar major depression is required before firm conclusions can be drawn regarding the familiality of major depression with psychotic features.

Cognitive Symptoms

Recently, research has found that PMDs, as compared with NPMDs and healthy controls, have greater deficits in various tests of cognition.[31] The most consistently replicated findings have been deficits in executive functioning,[31–36] verbal declarative memory,[31–33,37] and attention.[32,33,38] In addition, some studies have found deficits in response inhibition,[31] verbal story learning,[35] and visual-spatial perception and memory.[32,34]

As discussed in Gomez et al.,[33] there does not appear to be a generalized deficit in PMDs, but they perform worse than NPMDs and healthy controls on specific tasks. Importantly, PMDs have been found to have intact simple attention, which suggests that PMDs' ability to attend passively to units of information is within normal limits. However, they have more difficulty in processing, manipulating, and encoding new information. Furthermore, in a recent review and meta-analysis that included five available neuropsychological studies of PMDs,[39] the greatest cognitive deficits of PMDs compared with NPMDs were observed in verbal memory, executive functioning, and psychomotor speed. An issue that remains with this work is the medication status of the PMD patients because these patients are likely to have been exposed to, if they were not currently taking, antipsychotic medications, and it is unclear what effect this may have on cognition.

An earlier study by our group reported similar deficits in unmedicated PMDs compared with NPMDs and controls.[31] A recent study attempted to circumvent this medication problem and examined first-episode PMD, schizoaffective disorder, and schizophrenia patients, none of whom had been exposed to antipsychotic medication, and compared them with nonpsychotic unipolar depression (not first episode) and healthy controls.[34] They reported neuropsychological differences between the groups, including between the psychotic and nonpsychotic depressed patients. The authors concluded that "the data not only provide additional support for psychotic depression as a distinct mood disorder (from nonpsychotic depression) but also document the considerable neuropsychological morbidity associated with the disorder." They further found significant similarities between the neuropsychological profiles of the schizophrenic and psychotic depressed groups, suggesting that similar brain systems may be affected in both these disorders. Thus, there appears to be ample evidence for distinct neuropsychological profiles between PMD and NPMD, although limited research suggests that PMDs may be more similar to but slightly less severe than those with other psychotic disorders.

Biological Features

Patients with PMD have highly replicable findings of greater hypothalamic pituitary adrenal axis (HPA) activation: high rates of nonsuppression on the dexamethasone suppression test (DST), elevated post-dexamethasone cortisol levels, and high levels of 24-hour urinary free cortisol.[40–43] These findings are not just due to difference in the severity of the depression.[44,45] In addition, Anton[40] found that it was the older PMD patients who had the highest cortisol levels, suggesting an interaction between age and type of depression. We recently found that those depressed patients with psychotic features had higher evening baseline cortisol levels.[46] Furthermore, Rothschild et al.[42] compared four P.M. post-dexamethasone cortisol levels in PMD patients to those with schizophrenia and healthy controls. They found higher afternoon cortisol levels in PMD patients but not in those with schizophrenia. They concluded that the high cortisol levels were not due to psychosis per se, but rather to the presence of psychosis in the context of an affective disorder. Hence, there appears to be even greater HPA axis activity in PMD than in NPMD.

In pooled analyses, psychotic major depressives appear to have higher rates of nonsuppression on the DST and very elevated post-dexamethasone cortisol levels[41]: DST nonsuppression rates in PMD are about 64%, significantly higher than the 41% seen in NPMD. The sensitivity and specificity of the DST in PMD, however, are not high enough to be used routinely for diagnosis. Some studies, albeit generally small in size, even failed to show differences in nonsuppression rates between the two depressed groups.[41]

Other biological aspects of PMD have also been investigated. For example, PMD has been associated with a significant decrease in serum dopamine-beta-hydroxylase activity compared with controls, whereas NPMDs did not differ from controls[47] and with more rapid eye movement sleep disturbances compared with NPMD.[48] Structural and functional brain differences have also been found in PMDs compared with NPMDs and healthy controls. A number of years ago, Rothschild et al.[10] reported enlarged ventricles in computer tomography in PMD patients compared with NPMD patients, an observation replicated by some groups[49] but not by others.[50] Some of these earlier samples combine unipolar and bipolar psychotic depressed patients, which may lead to some of these inconsistent biological findings.

Treatment Response

Treatment response has also been found dependent on depression subtype. Dubvosky[51] concluded that about half of the depressed patients refractory to antidepressants have delusions and/or hallucinations of which the treating physician is unaware. Once, however, psychosis is detected, PMD patients still have different responses to the standard treatments. PMD is typically more difficult to treat than NPMD. Traditionally, it has been thought that electroconvulsive therapy (ECT) is more effective for PMD than for NPMD.[52,53] The results for relapse rate after ECT between PMD and NPMD are more variable. Some have found that PMDs have a higher relapse rate than NPMDs,[54,55] while others find no differences.[56] Prudic et al.[57] found that, in a community setting, remission rates for full courses of ECT were 30.3%–46.7% and that relapse was more frequent in patients with PMD. That study was open label, thus almost certainly overstating treatment response. More recently, Birkenhager and colleagues[58,59] found that among patients who had responded to ECT, those with psychotic depression relapsed less frequently than those with nonpsychotic depression. Tsuchiyama et al.[60] tried predicting who would respond to ECT but did not find that the presence of psychotic features contributed to the variance. Thus, although ECT may be effective in initially treating psychotic depression, the data are unclear regarding the duration of this effect in psychotic depression.

Historically, tricyclic antidepressant monotherapy was thought to be relatively ineffective in PMD compared with NPMD, with the former requiring a combination of antidepressants and antipsychotics. It has been generally thought that selective serotonin reuptake inhibitors (SSRIs) and serotonin and norepinephrine reuptake inhibitors as monotherapy would be similarly ineffective. One group has reported unexpectedly higher rates of response on monotherapy with SSRIs, but these studies have not been conducted under placebo-controlled conditions.[61–63] More recently, Rothschild et al.[64] examined the efficacy of olanzapine, placebo, or the combination of fluoxetine plus olanzapine in the treatment of PMD in two separate, parallel trials. In one trial, they found that, after 8 weeks of treatment, the group given combination therapy had greater improvement than did the group given placebo. In a second study, there were no significant differences in clinical outcome between the three treatment groups. Taken together, the combination separated from placebo first at 4 weeks and this difference continued out to 8 weeks. Although Howland[65] concluded that combining antidepressant and antipsychotic medications is the best approach if ECT is not used, this too remains uncertain. Interestingly, Rassmussen et al.[66] conducted a retrospective review of ECT and prior medication use. They found that among patients with psychotic depression, 95% had been given an inadequate combination of an antidepressant and antipsychotic agent, mostly due to low doses of the latter class. Similarly, Andreescu et al.[67] found that clinicians persistently use low doses of antipsychotics in the treatment of PMD. Thus, it is unclear whether ECT is truly more effective than drug therapy in PMD or whether patients are not adequately medicated. Overall, however, major depressive disorder (MDD) patients with psychotic features are clearly more difficult to treat effectively.

Overall, there are considerable data to indicate that psychotic depression is distinct from nonpsychotic depression in terms of clinical symptoms and course, biology, treatment response, and outcomes. However, there are inconsistencies among studies, and these measures may not be strong enough to be used in diagnosis. Thus, one could argue that more research is required before we adopt a designation of PMD as a separate disorder. Still the importance of psychotic features vis-à-vis clinical symptoms, course, and treatment in many studies does suggest that proper designation has a significant impact on outcome. Thus, whether one designates it as a separate disorder may be less important than developing better methods for delineating those patients with likely psychotic features to better guide care. Issues involved in this approach are described below.

Revamping the Current Diagnostic System

There are a number of issues that need to be considered even if one does not develop a separate designation for psychotic depression. First, in the current classification system, the presence of psychotic features is inexplicably linked to severity of depression. Second, the psychotic features' specifier is inadequately defined. What should be included—hallucinations or delusions only? What about cognitive disturbances such as odd thinking and poor cognitive function that are frequently observed, yet are not addressed, within the diagnosis? We believe that going to a dimensional system of psychotic symptoms or cognitive disturbance that is not linked to or dependent on severity would ultimately be more effective than the current binary classification of present or absent.

Psychosis Versus Severity

In the current *Diagnostic and Statistical Manual of Mental Disorders,* 4th Edition (DSM-IV)[68] classification of mood disorders, psychotic depression is described by a severity dimension specifier for major depressive episode, "severe with psychotic features." There is no way to designate a mild or moderate depression with psychotic features. However, research has shown that the relationship of severity and psychosis is not that strong. Ohayon and Schatzberg[5] reported that although the most severe forms of depression (as evidenced by meeting eight or nine of the nine DSM depression criteria) were associated with higher rates of psychosis (33%), those with mild to moderate major depression also demonstrated relatively high rates of psychosis (15% and higher). Furthermore, they found that those with specific symptoms, particularly feelings of worthlessness and guilt, were most likely to have psychotic features; however, the severity of these two symptoms was not associated with the presence of psychotic features. In another recent study carried out in a large sample of patients with an index episode of major depression, Maj et al.[18] found that the index episode was more likely to be severe in patients with psychotic versus nonpsychotic depression but that in 23.6% of patients with psychotic depression the index episode was either mild or moderate. On the other hand, many severely depressed patients do not develop psychotic features.[13,69] Thus, severity of depression alone does not entirely account for the presence of psychotic symptoms.

One recommendation to address this issue is to separate the dimensions of severity and psychosis. The severity dimension would continue to consist of 1 = mild, 2 = moderate, and 3 = severe, and a separate dimension would then take into account psychotic symptoms. The question then becomes: how do we characterize a dimension of psychosis? There are a number of ways in which this could be done. Above, we have reviewed the clinical and cognitive symptoms of psychotic depression. Below we discuss the clinical and cognitive symptoms of psychotic depression and how they may be incorporated into a psychosis dimension.

Psychotic and Cognitive Symptoms

Clinically, it is important to note that the boundary between psychotic and nonpsychotic symptoms is not always clearly delineated. Thoughts (or feelings) of guilt, worthlessness, deserved punishment, physical disease, poverty, and nihilism may be present in various degrees in depressed patients, with fluctuations within the same episode. Maj et al.[18] found that, out of 452 patients with an index episode of major depression, 19.7% had at least one belief fulfilling both DSM-IV prerequisites for delusions, while 27.2% had no delusion but at least one sustained preoccupation, including 5.3% who met one of the DSM-IV prerequisites for delusions but not the other (i.e., the belief was of "delusional proportions" but was not maintained with "delusional intensity," or vice versa). How persistent the delusional quality must be in order to justify the diagnosis of psychotic depression is at present unclear. The same applies to hallucinations, which in several cases occur only occasionally, whose perceptual quality may not be straightforward and whose distinction from illusions (i.e., misperceptions, colored by the depressed mood, of real sounds or voices) may be imprecise.

Guilt and feelings of worthlessness are two items that particularly fall into this category. For example, guilt is a common symptom of depression, and it may be best seen on a continuum of behavior rather than categorical present or absent. In many cases, the guilt may be beyond what is typically expected in depression but yet may not be fully delusional. A dimensional model of the psychotic specifier would account for such ambiguous symptoms.

The DSM-IV distinction between mood-congruent and mood-incongruent psychotic symptoms in depressed patients makes intuitive sense; however, there is little specific evidence for this distinction or its relevance. Mood congruence may be difficult to evaluate in some cases, and both mood-congruent and mood-incongruent symptoms may be present at the same time.[18,70] In some studies, the presence of mood-incongruent psychotic symptoms in depressed patients was a predictor of a poorer outcome, but other studies did not replicate this finding.[71,72] It would be advisable in DSM-V to allow to record at the same time both mood-congruent and mood-incongruent psychotic symptoms or to use the expression "with predominant" mood-congruent or mood-incongruent psychotic symptoms. Further research is needed to understand the prognostic implications of these specific symptoms and the mood-congruent/incongruent psychotic distinction.

We propose that one way to assess psychosis is to develop dimensional ratings for specific psychotic as well as cognitive symptoms. One dimension could describe reality distortions from a mild UTC to frank delusions; another dimension would describe cognitive impairment that would encompass difficulties such as memory or concentration problems. Thus, one dimension would be used to assess psychosis/odd thinking/changes in reality with a scale from 0=not present, 1=vague, ideas of reference that are largely mood congruent, 2=unusual thought patterns (not part of a delusion, not fixed thinking, or frequent illusions), 3=subthreshold delusion, not quite fixed beliefs, and 4=fixed, misperception of reality (fully delusional) or definite presence of hallucinations. The second dimensional scale could cover cognitive processes/thinking. This dimension would likely be based on formal cognitive testing, which would encompass the domains that have been found to be impaired in PMDs, such as executive functioning, memory, and psychomotor speed. More research is necessary to determine which specific tests could be utilized in such a battery, and it would be necessary that such a battery is quickly and easily administered and has good sensitivity and specificity to psychotic depression. Here the ranges are less clear but could be rated as a scale from 0=no cognitive impairment, 1=impairment of one domain, 2=impairment of two domains, and 3=impairment of three domains, such that higher number indicates more domain impairment. For this dimension, we feel it would be important to have a short, standard battery to administer because very often depressed patients will have subjective cognitive complaints in the absence of quantitative deficits.

Relationship to Bipolar and Schizoaffective Disorder

A relationship between psychotic unipolar, major depression, and bipolar disorder has been repeatedly suggested on the basis of family history and risk of conversion.[28] There is considerable evidence to suggest that PMD is likely to represent a first episode of a bipolar disorder in younger patients. Because young patients often have less in the way of a history of mood problems, they may not have yet experienced the necessary hypomania or mania for a bipolar diagnosis at the time of their first depressive episode. For example, as noted above, Maj et al.[18] found that the switch to bipolarity was significantly associated with an earlier first psychiatric contact and a family history of bipolar I disorder but not with the presence of delusions in the index episode. Incidentally, many young, psychotic depressives do not convert to bipolar in a 10-year follow-up. It is clear that the issue of the overlap between PMD and bipolar disorder warrants further research attention in all the domains discussed above.

There is some difficulty distinguishing between psychotic depression and schizoaffective disorder, particularly in early episodes. In part, this occurs because the course and history of the depressive and psychotic symptoms are key to making an appropriate diagnosis. There is less history available in early episodes. Schizoaffective disorder tends to be chronic with a chronic thought disorder even when the patient is not depressed, whereas psychotic depression, including any thought disorder, is episodic. However, there are some similarities. As noted earlier, there is evidence to suggest that cognitive deficits in PMD may be more similar to but slightly less severe than those with schizoaffective disorder.[34] Furthermore, there is some evidence that long-term outcome for schizoaffective disorder patients is more similar to affective disorders than to schizophrenia.[73] The potential overlap between PMD and schizoaffective disorder warrants further research attention.

Conclusions

In conclusion, currently available research evidence supports the usefulness of some "psychosis" specifier in the diagnosis of major depression. This specifier should be kept separate from the "severity" one. It should be possible to record the presence of both mood-congruent and mood-incongruent psychotic features in the same patient. More precise guidelines should be provided about how to distinguish psychotic from nonpsychotic experiences (e.g., delusional from nondelusional guilt and hallucinations from illusions). These should highlight how persistent experiences need to be in order to justify a label of psychosis. Some biological findings could be acknowledged in the "Associated Laboratory Findings" section of DSM, but the diagnostic criteria should be based on the clinical picture.

There are a number of research areas that could help address the needs laid out for psychotic depression categorization. First, it would be important to consider the definition of psychosis in the context of major depression. Does the definition need to be broadened to include cognitive distortions, not just full delusions? What are the primary delusions that occur in PMD? How should these be defined and what distortions are commonly seen in the context of MDD?

Formal thought disorder in severely depressed patients is understudied. The BPRS conceptual disorganization item is perhaps not optimal to explore this disorder because it is framed on the formal thought disorder of schizophrenia and is but one item. One characteristic of the formal thought disorder of depressed patients is that, contrary to what is assumed by the BPRS, its quality is not necessarily reflected by the degree of verbal production. For instance, a severely depressed patient with crowded or racing thoughts will often have a reduced (rather than increased) verbal production based on the nature of the mood component. Thus, we do not know whether, to what extent, or how formal thought disorder is manifest in major depression nor do we know its relationship to formal thought disorder in schizophrenia. More specific research in this area is warranted.

The DSM-IV distinction between mood-congruent and mood-incongruent psychotic symptoms in depressed patients makes intuitive sense. However, there is little specific evidence for this distinction or its relevance. It would be helpful to gather more data on the prevalence and importance of mood congruence in relation to prognosis, course, and outcome. Other issues to be investigated include: does having mood-incongruent psychotic symptoms put one at greater risk for relapse or a manic episode? Do those with mood-congruent psychotic symptoms have a better outcome than those with mood-incongruent symptoms?

A second important area of research is to develop a short neurocognitive battery that could help differentiate PMD from NPMD. Neurocognitive batteries can be very complex and time consuming, and these would not be of benefit within a typical clinical practice. However, if a short battery could be developed to differentiate these patients with adequate sensitivity and specificity, it would be a very useful clinical tool. Starting with the neuropsychological findings to date, executive functioning, verbal memory, and psychomotor speed are the three areas that consistently are found to be impaired in PMDs. Issues that remain problematic within the neuropsychology of PMD are that there are relatively few studies and that medication status can be a factor.

A third issue for further study is whether any of the clinical, cognitive, or biological variables discussed above have diagnostic or prognostic value for psychotic depression. For example, do any of the specific psychotic or cognitive symptoms predict future PMD episodes or time to remission in the current episode? We already know that the presence of delusions and hallucinations in depressed patients does have some prognostic implications. Does the severity of the depressive episode (mild, moderate, or severe) also play a role in outcome? Psychotic episodes tend to have a longer duration and the recurrence rate tends to be higher. However, the medium- and long-term prognostic implications are less clear. In several studies, there was no significant difference in the outcome at 7 or 10 years between depressed patients with mood-congruent psychotic symptoms and nonpsychotic depressives. This may be in part due to the fact, reported by Winokur et al.,[74] that psychotic symptoms tend to become less prominent late in the course of the illness. This finding, however, requires replication.

In addition, data suggest that the presence of delusions and hallucinations in depressed patients has therapeutic implications. Depressed patients with mood-congruent delusions and hallucinations are less likely to respond to antidepressant monotherapy than nonpsychotic depressives, but this is largely based on the tricyclic literature. However, the Italian data are highly suggestive of a potential benefit with SSRI monotherapy. This requires further controlled data.

There is some overlap between unipolar psychotic depression and bipolar disorder. A family history of bipolar disorder is significantly more frequent in depressed patients with mood-congruent psychotic symptoms than in nonpsychotic depressives, and we found that the percentage of patients with at least two manic symptoms in their index episode was significantly higher in the former.[18] The prognostic and therapeutic implications of these findings should be further explored. Data on the familiality of psychotic depression is also needed to better understand genetic influences. Furthermore, we do not have adequate data on cognitive and biological overlap of PMD and bipolar disorder, and this may warrant further investigation. Last, the clinical, biological, and treatment differentiation between PMD and schizoaffective disorder (depressed type) needs further study as well.

References

1. Blazer DG, Kessler RC, McGonagle KA, Swartz MS. The prevalence and distribution of major depression in a national community sample: the National Comorbidity Survey. Am J Psychiatry. 1994;151:979–986.
2. Jenkins R, Lewis G, Bebbington P, et al. The National Psychiatric Morbidity surveys of Great Britain—initial findings from the household survey. Psychol Med. 1997;27:775–789.
3. Oakley-Browne MA, Joyce PR, Wells JE, Bushnell JA, Hornblow AR. Christchurch Psychiatric Epidemiology Study, Part II: six month and other period prevalences of specific psychiatric disorders. Aust N Z J Psychiatry. 1989;23:327–340.
4. Weissman MM, Bland RC, Canino GJ, et al. Cross-national epidemiology of major depression and bipolar disorder. JAMA. 1996;276:293–299.

5. Ohayon MM, Schatzberg AF. Prevalence of depressive episodes with psychotic features in the general population. Am J Psychiatry. 2002;159:1855–1861.
6. Roy A. Hypothalamic-pituitary-adrenal axis function and suicidal behavior in depression. Biol Psychiatry. 1992;32:812–816.
7. Johnson J, Horwath E, Weissman MM. The validity of major depression with psychotic features based on a community study. Arch Gen Psychiatry. 1991;48:1075–1081.
8. Rothschild AJ. Challenges in the treatment of depression with psychotic features. Biol Psychiatry. 2003;53:680–690.
9. Schatzberg AF, Rothschild AJ. Psychotic (delusional) major depression: should it be included as a distinct syndrome in DSM-IV? Am J Psychiatry. 1992;149:733–745.
10. Rothschild AJ, Benes F, Hebben N, et al. Relationships between brain CT scan findings and cortisol in psychotic and nonpsychotic depressed patients. Biol Psychiatry. 1989;26:565–575.
11. Charney DS, Nelson JC. Delusional and nondelusional unipolar depression: further evidence for distinct subtypes. Am J Psychiatry. 1981;138:328–333.
12. Lykouras E, Malliaras D, Christodoulou GN, et al. Delusional depression: phenomenology and response to treatment: a prospective study. Acta Psychiatr Scand. 1986;73:324–329.
13. Glassman AH, Roose SP. Delusional depression: a distinct clinical entity? Arch Gen Psychiatry. 1981;138:831–833.
14. Parker G, Hadzi-Pavlovic D, Hickie I, et al. Distinguishing psychotic and non-psychotic melancholia. J Affect Disord. 1991;22:135–148.
15. Keller J, Gomez RG, Kenna HA, et al. Detecting psychotic major depression using psychiatric rating scales. J Psychiatr Res. 2006;40:22–29.
16. Overall JE, Gorham DE. The brief psychiatric rating scale. Psychol Rep. 1961;10:799–812.
17. Coryell W, Endicott J, Keller M. The importance of psychotic features to major depression: course and outcome during a 2-year follow-up. Acta Psychiatr Scand. 1987;75:78–85.
18. Maj M, Pirozzi R, Magliano L, Fiorillo A, Bartoli L. Phenomenology and prognostic significance of delusions in major depressive disorder: a 10-year follow-up study. J Clin Psychiatry. 2007;68:1411–1417.
19. Aronson TA, Shukla S, Gujavarty K, Hoff A, DiBuono M, Khan E. Relapse in delusional depression: a retrospective study of the course of treatment. Compr Psychiatry. 1988;29:12–21.
20. Nelson JC, Bowers MB Jr. Delusional unipolar depression: description and drug response. Arch Gen Psychiatry. 1978;35:1321–1328.
21. Black DW, Winokur G, Nasrallah A. Effect of psychosis on suicide risk in 1,593 patients with unipolar and bipolar affective disorders. Am J Psychiatry. 1988;145:849–852.
22. Vythilingam M, Chen J, Bremner JD, Mazure CM, Maciejewski PK, Nelson JC. Psychotic depression and mortality. Am J Psychiatry. 2003;160:574–576.
23. Coryell W, Tsuang MT. Primary unipolar depression and the prognostic importance of delusions. Arch Gen Psychiatry. 1982;39:1181–1184.
24. Kassem L, Lopez V, Hedeker D, Steele J, Zandi P, McMahon FJ. Familiality of polarity at illness onset in bipolar affective disorder. Am J Psychiatry. 2006;163:1754–1759.

25. Pardo PJ, Knesevich MA, Vogler GP, et al. Genetic and state variables of neurocognitive dysfunction in schizophrenia: a twin study. Schizophr Bull. 2000;26:459–477.

26. Leckman JF, Weissman MM, Prusoff BA, et al. Subtypes of depression. Family study perspective. Arch Gen Psychiatry. 1984;41:833–838.

27. Nelson WH, Khan A, Orr WW Jr. Delusional depression. Phenomenology, neuroendocrine function, and tricyclic antidepressant response. J Affect Disord. 1984;6:297–306.

28. Weissman MM, Prusoff BA, Merikangas KR. Is delusional depression related to bipolar disorder? Am J Psychiatry. 1984;141:892–893.

29. Akiskal HS, Walker P, Puzantian VR, King D, Rosenthal TL, Dranon M. Bipolar outcome in the course of depressive illness. Phenomenologic, familial, and pharmacologic predictors. J Affect Disord. 1983;5:115–128.

30. Strober M, Carlson G. Bipolar illness in adolescents with major depression: clinical, genetic, and psychopharmacologic predictors in a three- to four-year prospective follow-up investigation. Arch Gen Psychiatry. 1982;39:549–555.

31. Schatzberg AF, Posener JA, DeBattista C, Kalehzan BM, Rothschild AJ, Shear PK. Neuropsychological deficits in psychotic versus nonpsychotic major depression and no mental illness. Am J Psychiatry. 2000;157:1095–1100.

32. Basso MR, Bornstein RA. Neuropsychological deficits in psychotic versus nonpsychotic unipolar depression. Neuropsychology. 1999;13:69–75.

33. Gomez RG, Fleming SH, Keller J, et al. The neuropsychological profile of psychotic major depression and its relation to cortisol. Biol Psychiatry. 2006;60:472–478.

34. Hill SK, Keshavan MS, Thase ME, Sweeney JA. Neuropsychological dysfunction in antipsychotic-naive first-episode unipolar psychotic depression. Am J Psychiatry. 2004;161:996–1003.

35. Jeste DV, Heaton SC, Paulsen JS, Ercoli L, Harris J, Heaton RK. Clinical and neuropsychological comparison of psychotic depression with nonpsychotic depression and schizophrenia. Am J Psychiatry. 1996;153:490–496.

36. Nelson EB, Sax KW, Strakowski SM. Attentional performance in patients with psychotic and nonpsychotic major depression and schizophrenia. Am J Psychiatry. 1998;155:137–139.

37. Belanoff JK, Kalehzan M, Sund B, Fleming Ficek SK, Schatzberg AF. Cortisol activity and cognitive changes in psychotic major depression. Am J Psychiatry. 2001;158:1612–1616.

38. Kim DK, Kim BL, Sohn SE, et al. Candidate neuroanatomic substrates of psychosis in old-aged depression. Prog Neuropsychopharmacol Biol Psychiatry. 1999;23:793–807.

39. Fleming SK, Blasey C, Schatzberg AF. Neuropsychological correlates of psychotic features in major depressive disorders: a review and meta-analysis. J Psychiatr Res. 2004;38:27–35.

40. Anton RF. Urinary free cortisol in psychotic depression. Biol Psychiatry. 1987;22:24–34.

41. Nelson JC, Davis JM. DST studies in psychotic depression: a meta-analysis. Am J Psychiatry. 1997;154:1497–1503.

42. Rothschild AJ, Schatzberg AF, Rosenbaum AH, Stahl JB, Cole JO. The dexamethasone suppression test as a discriminator among subtypes of psychotic patients. Br J Psychiatry. 1982;141:471–474.

43. Schatzberg AF, Rothschild AJ, Stahl JB, et al. The dexamethasone suppression test: identification of subtypes of depression. Am J Psychiatry. 1983;140:88–91.

44. Brown RP, Stoll PM, Stokes PE, et al. Adrenocortical hyperactivity in depression: effects of agitation, delusions, melancholia, and other illness variables. Psychiatry Res. 1988;23:167–178.

45. Evans DL, Nemeroff CB. Use of the dexamethasone suppression test using DSM-III criteria on an inpatient psychiatric unit. Biol Psychiatry. 1983;18:505–511.

46. Keller J, Flores B, Gomez RG, et al. Cortisol circadian rhythm alterations in psychotic major depression. Biol Psychiatry. 2006;60:275–281.

47. Sapru MK, Rao BS, Channabasavanna SM. Serum dopamine- beta-hydroxylase activity in clinical subtypes of depression. Acta Psychiatr Scand. 1989;80:474–478.

48. Thase ME, Kupfer DJ, Ulrich RF. Electroencephalographic sleep in psychotic depression. A valid subtype? Arch Gen Psychiatry. 1986;43:886–893.

49. Targum SD, Rosen LN, DeLisi LE, Weinberger DR, Citrin CM. Cerebral ventricular size in major depressive disorder: association with delusional symptoms. Biol Psychiatry. 1983;18:329–336.

50. Luchins DJ, Meltzer HY. Ventricular size and psychosis in affective disorder. Biol Psychiatry. 1983;18:1197–1198.

51. Dubovsky SL. What we don't know about psychotic depression. Biol Psychiatry. 1991;30:533–536.

52. Buchan H, Johnstone E, McPherson K, Palmer RL, Crow TJ, Brandon S. Who benefits from electroconvulsive therapy? Combined results of the Leicester and Northwick Park trials. Br J Psychiatry. 1992;160:355–359.

53. Petrides G, Fink M, Husain MM, et al. ECT remission rates in psychotic versus non-psychotic depressed patients: a report from CORE. J ECT. 2001;17:244–253.

54. O'Leary DA, Lee AS. Seven year prognosis in depression. Mortality and readmission risk in the Nottingham ECT cohort. Br J Psychiatry. 1996;169:423–429.

55. Spiker DG, Stein J, Rich CL. Delusional depression and electroconvulsive therapy: one year later. Convuls Ther. 1985;1:167–172.

56. Sackeim HA, Prudic J, Devanand DP, Decina P, Kerr B, Malitz S. The impact of medication resistance and continuation pharmacotherapy on relapse following response to electroconvulsive therapy in major depression. J Clin Psychopharmacol. 1990;10:96–104.

57. Prudic J, Olfson M, Marcus SC, Fuller RB, Sackeim HA. Effectiveness of electroconvulsive therapy in community settings. Biol Psychiatry. 2004;55:301–312.

58. Birkenhager TK, Renes JW, Pluijms EM. One-year follow-up after successful ECT: a naturalistic study in depressed inpatients. J Clin Psychiatry. 2004;65:87–91.

59. Birkenhager TK, van den Broek WW, Mulder PG, de Lely A. One-year outcome of psychotic depression after successful electroconvulsive therapy. J ECT. 2005;21:221–226.

60. Tsuchiyama K, Nagayama H, Yamada K, Isogawa K, Katsuragi S, Kiyota A. Predicting efficacy of electroconvulsive therapy in major depressive disorder. Psychiatry Clin Neurosci. 2005;59:546–550.

61. Zanardi R, Franchini L, Gasperini M, Perez J, Smeraldi E. Double-blind controlled trial of sertraline versus paroxetine in the treatment of delusional depression. Am J Psychiatry. 1996;153:1631–1633.

62. Zanardi R, Franchini L, Gasperini M, Lucca A, Smeraldi E, Perez J. Faster onset of action of fluvoxamine in combination with pindolol in the treatment of delusional depression: a controlled study. J Clin Psychopharmacol. 1998;18:441–446.

63. Zanardi R, Franchini L, Serretti A, Perez J, Smeraldi E. Venlafaxine versus fluvoxamine in the treatment of delusional depression: a pilot double-blind controlled study. J Clin Psychiatry. 2000;61:26–29.

64. Rothschild AJ, Williamson DJ, Tohen MF, et al. A double-blind, randomized study of olanzapine and olanzapine/fluoxetine combination for major depression with psychotic features. J Clin Psychopharmacol. 2004;24:365–373.

65. Howland RH. Pharmacotherapy for psychotic depression. J Psychosoc Nurs Ment Health Serv. 2006;44:13–17.

66. Rasmussen KG, Mueller M, Kellner CH, et al. Patterns of psychotropic medication use among patients with severe depression referred for electroconvulsive therapy: data from the consortium for research on electroconvulsive therapy. J ECT. 2006;22:116–123.

67. Andreescu C, Mulsant BH, Peasley-Miklus C, et al. Persisting low use of antipsychotics in the treatment of major depressive disorder with psychotic features. J Clin Psychiatry. 2007;68:194–200.

68. American Psychiatric Association. Diagnostic and Statistical Manual of Mental Disorders. 4th ed. Washington, DC: American Psychiatric Association; 1994.

69. Endicott J, Spitzer RL. Use of the Research Diagnostic Criteria and the Schedule for Affective Disorders and Schizophrenia to study affective disorders. Am J Psychiatry. 1979;136:52–56.

70. Black DW, Nasrallah A. Hallucinations and delusions in 1,715 patients with unipolar and bipolar affective disorders. Psychopathology. 1989;22:28–34.

71. Coryell W, Tsuang MT. Major depression with mood-congruent or mood-incongruent psychotic features: outcome after 40 years. Am J Psychiatry. 1985;142:479–482.

72. Jäger M, Bottlender R, Strauss A, Möller HJ. Fifteen-year follow-up of Diagnostic and Statistical Manual of Mental Disorders, Fourth Edition depressive disorders: the prognostic significance of psychotic features. Compr Psychiatry. 2005;46:322–327.

73. Jäger M, Bottlender R, Strauss A, Möller HJ. Fifteen-year follow-up of ICD-10 schizoaffective disorders compared with schizophrenia and affective disorders. Acta Psychiatr Scand. 2004;109:30–37.

74. Winokur G, Scharfetter C, Angst J. Stability of psychotic symptomatology (delusions, hallucinations), affective syndromes, and schizophrenic symptoms (thought disorder, incongruent affect) over episodes in remitting psychoses. Eur Arch Psychiatry Neurol Sci. 1985;234:303–307.

4

DECONSTRUCTING BIPOLAR DISORDER

A Critical Review of Its Diagnostic Validity and a Proposal for DSM-V and ICD-11

Eduard Vieta, M.D., Ph.D.
Mary L. Phillips, M.D., MRCPsych

Introduction

CHALLENGING THE KRAEPELINIAN DICHOTOMY: CATEGORICAL VERSUS DIMENSIONAL APPROACHES

Modern classifications of mental disorders assume a categorical model that may be helpful in terms of reliability and communication among clinicians and researchers, but which raises serious concerns about diagnostic validity and boundaries between entities. The concept of psychosis and the entities that may be grouped under that umbrella may themselves be questionable. Moreover, the classification of psychoses has been a topic of vigorous debate ever since its conception with the formulation of

Reprinted with permission from Vieta E, Phillips ML. "Deconstructing Bipolar Disorder: A Critical Review of Its Diagnostic Validity and a Proposal for DSM-V and ICD-11." *Schizophrenia Bulletin* 2007; 33: 886–892.

Supported in part by the National Institutes of Health (NIH) grant for the conference titled "Deconstructing Psychosis" convened under the auspices of the American Psychiatric Association, the World Health Organization, and the NIH in Washington, DC, February 15–17, 2006.

the disease concepts of dementia praecox and manic-depressive insanity by Emil Kraepelin in 1896 and their subsequent codification into the nosological entities of schizophrenia and bipolar illness.[1,2] There has been an intensive debate on whether these two conditions are distinct or related and potentially overlapping illnesses. Categorical approaches, as those from *Diagnostic and Statistical Manual of Mental Disorders,* 4th Edition, Text Revision (DSM-IV-TR),[3] and *International Classification of Diseases,* 10th Edition (ICD-10),[4] may be useful in clinical practice but leave many patients out of the diagnostic system (the disappointing subcategory of "not otherwise specified") and provide a very poor solution to the problem of symptomatic overlap, either by causing huge comorbidity or by creating intermediate categories such as "schizoaffective disorder." From the research point of view, dimensional approaches seem much more useful but are clearly less practical under routine clinical conditions.

THE VALIDITY OF PSYCHIATRIC DIAGNOSIS

In the absence of an etiologically based classification, attempts have been made to build a diagnostic system of mental conditions that could be used across different cultures. As formulated by Robins and Guze,[5] introducing a biomedical approach to psychiatric nosology that has been extremely successful in the last three decades, the validity of psychiatric diagnosis may rely on several domains: 1) content validity, involving basically symptoms and clinical diagnostic criteria; 2) concurrent validity, defined by neurobiological correlates such as laboratory findings, neuroimaging and neuropsychology, genetics, family studies, and perhaps also treatment response; 3) predictive validity, which has mainly to do with diagnostic stability over time; and 4) discriminant validity, which involves delimitation from other disorders. This formulation, directly inherited from Sydenham's approach to general medicine, had the virtue of approaching psychiatry to other medical specialties. It also allowed to counteract the predominant Freudian theories that were leaving psychiatry orphan of any operational taxonomy, and it became the foundation of the first modern classification of psychiatric disorders based on operationalized criteria (St. Louis[6]), and the grounds for the most successful one (DSM-III[7]). Further developments were DSM-III-R,[8] DSM-IV,[9] and DSM-IV-TR. In 1992, The World Health Organization applied the same approach to their latter version of ICD-10.[4]

The Validity of Bipolar Disorder as a Diagnostic Category

CONTENT VALIDITY PROBLEMS OF CURRENT DEFINITIONS OF BIPOLAR DISORDER

The concept of bipolar disorder involves the current or past occurrence of at least one episode of mania or hypomania or a mixed episode, which is usually, but not necessarily, preceded or followed by a depressive episode, cyclic changes between mood states, and eventually psychotic symptoms, which are assumed to be a marker of the severity of the episode. By excluding psychotic symptoms from the definition, leaving them as mere correlate of impairment or severity (criterion D), DSMs have indirectly reinforced the (wrong) idea that psychotic symptoms are a core feature of schizophrenia but not bipolar disorder. Furthermore, they have taken little advantage of the potential value of characterizing psychotic features (i.e., mood congruent vs. mood incongruent) for discriminant validity versus schizophrenia.

Moreover, the definition of major depression in bipolar disorder in DSM does not make any difference with unipolar depression. Nevertheless, DSM acknowledges the bipolar/unipolar dichotomy as opposed to the Kraepelinian concept of manic-depressive illness, which is still advocated by some authors.[10] This carries the problem that the diagnosis of bipolar depression can only be made after a manic, hypomanic, or mixed episode has occurred. The system is, thus, assuming some loss of predictive validity in unipolar depression and increasing the heterogeneity of the concept of major depression, which may be too broad. Conversely, the concept of mixed episodes is very narrowly defined as the concurrence of a full manic and depressive episode, leaving behind many potentially useful concepts such as mixed hypomania[11,12] and excluding the possibility that bipolar II patients may have mixed episodes. The definition of mixed states underlines once again the difficulties of converting dimensional concepts into diagnostic categories.

ICD-10 was to ICD-9[13] what DSM-III was to DSM-II[14]: a major switch from a pure classification code toward a novel classification with operational diagnostic criteria; in some way, it was born as a "global" alternative to DSM-III. As far as bipolar disorder is concerned, the most relevant difference between the two systems is that in ICD-10 episodes are also diagnoses and that hypomania is seen as mild form of mania in the latter (1 week duration, social impairment needed); to differentiate the concept between affective and nonaffective psychoses, the "prominence" of psychotic versus affective symptoms is claimed, without any clear definition of what prominence means.

CONCURRENT VALIDITY: THE NEED OF EMBEDDING BIOLOGICAL MARKERS INTO THE DIAGNOSTIC SYSTEM

To a great extent, the social success of medicine over the past 100 years has depended on laboratory findings and the support of technology to clinician's skills. In psychiatry, practically no tools other than psychopathological assessment are still available as routine diagnostic tests, and in fact, this is one of the main reasons why a reliable, clinically based diagnostic system is still necessary, but there has been substantial progress in using biological findings as diagnostic validators. Hence, the list of findings in bipolar disorder with significantly better sensitivity and specificity than chance is quite long, but none of them has a clear use in clinical practice.

However, the coming diagnostic systems cannot ignore anymore this long list of validators, including laboratory, neuroimaging, neuropsychology, genetic, and therapeutic data. Therefore, it may be the time to design a "psychiatric toolbox," including genotyping, neurophysiological, neuroimaging, and neuropsychological tests, which may help to identify biomarkers that are persistent, rather than trait dependent, to improve the validity of the psychiatric classification and its pathophysiological grounds. Clearly, more research is urgently needed in order to be able, as soon as possible, to add laboratory measures to the classification system.

Although concurrent validity can be narrowly defined to include only "hard" laboratory data, we think that family studies, which were defined separately by Robins and Guze,[5] and neuropsychological findings can be included in this concept too. There is no question that the exclusion of family data from the diagnostic systems was not decided merely on sensitivity/specificity ratio; in fact, family history may be much more useful for certain conditions, including bipolar disorder, than some of the official criteria in the DSM-IV list. It was rather a "philosophical" decision, which should be revised promptly. Assuming that there is no single symptom that is exclusive of bipolar disorder or schizophrenia, including the Schneiderian first-rank symptoms,[15] the utility of family history is probably higher than that of many of the current criteria.

With regard to genetics, current knowledge supports that there is indeed some overlap in the genes that predispose to bipolar disorder and schizophrenia. One gene, *(G72),* has been repeatedly implicated as an overlap gene,[16] whereas *DISC1, COMT, BDNF,* and others may constitute additional shared susceptibility genes.[17] However, potential nonoverlap syndromes—such as nonpsychotic bipolar disorder or cyclothymia on the one hand, and negative symptoms or the deficit syndrome on the other—could turn out to have their own unique genetic determinants.[18] If genotypes are to be the anchor points of a clinically useful system of classification, they must ultimately be shown to inform prognosis, treatment, and prevention. No gene variants have yet met these tests in bipolar disorder or schizophrenia but may, it is hoped, be used as diagnostic validators concurrently with clinical criteria in the near future.

Imaging data examining volume loss in brain structures are also consistent with some overlap between diagnostic categories within the spectrum of psychoses. Genetic risk for schizophrenia may be associated with volume loss in gray matter in left frontal-striatum–thalamic and temporal areas, whereas the genetic risk for bipolar disorder may be associated with volume loss in gray matter in the right anterior cingulate cortex and in the ventral striatum. However, genetic risk for both conditions is also associated with brain changes as volume loss in white matter in frontal and temporoparietal areas.[19] The most prominent brain abnormality in bipolar disorder is enlargement of the amygdala.[20] In addition, there might be structural changes in other limbic structures and hippocampus, the frontal lobe, cerebellum, and pituitary.[21] Again, none of these findings is specific enough to be used as a diagnostic test in clinical practice, but the consistency of the findings suggests that they do have some diagnostic validity. As an example of the progress made by neuroimaging studies in particular in providing data to support the diagnostic validity of bipolar disorder, we discuss in Chapter 10, "Identifying Functional Neuroimaging Biomarkers of Bipolar Disorder," recent promising findings from structural and functional neuroimaging studies that suggest persistent regional neural abnormalities in bipolar disorder.

Neuropsychological tests have shown consistently that both schizophrenia and bipolar disorder are associated with significant cognitive problems, which may be more intense in the former.[22,23] Differences may involve attention, verbal memory, and executive function[24] and particularly premorbid intelligence.[25–27] None of these issues is currently included in the classificatory system. Some of the reasons that are often given to exclude this kind of information from the diagnostic criteria are that their specificity is not very high and they are not available to the majority of clinicians. However, this could be easily solved by devoting a supplementary axis to biological and neuropsychological markers, which could, initially, work just as a source of complementary or supportive information that might also help to stimulate further research.

Indeed, there is a long-lasting tradition in psychiatry to try to use laboratory tests to verify clinical impressions. The initial expectations related to rapid eye movement (REM) latency tests and dexamethasone suppression tests were not accomplished because they would not be able to replace clinical judgment, and actually their sensitivity/specificity ratio was poorer than that of most clinical criteria used in the classificatory system. Subsequently, many other neurophysiological and biochemical tests have been developed, showing consistently that bipolar disorder has significant neurobiological correlates that may enhance concurrent validity, as suggested in our proposal for a modular classification below.

Biomarkers may increase not only concurrent validity but also discriminant validity. The same applies to treatment response. In the case of bipolar disorder, treatment response may be particularly helpful as far as lithium and perhaps other so-called mood stabilizers are concerned: Lithium has been reported to be effective in mania but not in schizophrenia[28] and is likely to be more effective in bipolar depression than unipolar depression.[29] Lamotrigine may also be more helpful for bipolar depression than unipolar depression.[30] There may be a familial disposition to lithium response.[31] Bipolar patients are also more likely to switch to mania when treated with antidepressants than unipolar patients.[32]

DISCRIMINANT VALIDITY OF BIPOLAR DISORDER: DELIMITATION FROM OTHER DISORDERS

In the absence of an etiological classification, discriminant validity is far from ideal in any classification. Symptom overlap is huge in psychiatry, and differences between conditions are more quantitative than qualitative. This is one of the reasons why dimensional approaches may be much more valid, albeit less practical, than categorical. The problems of a categorical classification in a dimensional world are as follows: 1) many patients do not fit in any category (due to artificial boundaries and "holes" between them); 2) many patients do not achieve enough severity or duration of symptoms to qualify for the full picture, despite suffering from similar consequences as those with the whole syndrome (spectrum); and 3) many patients fulfill criteria for several conditions because of symptom overlap (comorbidity). The only way that DSM-IV, ICD-10, and similar systems have found to cope with problems related to discriminant validity as those mentioned above has been to allow for switching within categories (i.e., unipolar to bipolar after a manic episode) to include broad categories as "not otherwise specified," the inclusion of milder categories within a spectrum (i.e., bipolar II), and to allow for coexistence of several diagnosis within the same patient (comorbidity). However, and challenging the statement that these classifications are atheoretical, some particular comorbidities are not allowed: for instance, the apparent dilemma of allowing the co-occurrence of the two major psychoses, schizophrenia and manic-depressive illness, in the same patient is solved with the introduction of another intermediate category, schizoaffective disorder, which has poor content validity and reliability but helps to avoid the problem. Conversely, some patients may happen to fulfill criteria for more than 10 different conditions, a phenomenon that does not happen in any other medical specialty.

Laboratory data have been disappointing with regard to support boundaries between conditions; they seem to behave as symptoms, with important overlap and poor specificity. There are some emerging data from neuroimaging studies, though, pointing to bipolar-specific regional neural functional abnormalities (reviewed in Chapter 10). Again, however, genetics, neuropathology, neurophysiology, neuroimaging, biochemical challenge tests, and neuropsychology, while providing some support to diagnostic boundaries, are unable to work at present as diagnostic tests in clinical practice. But even if we are not there yet, the preliminary inclusion of laboratory data to support to some extent the validity of either categories or dimensions may carry more benefits than problems. In the future, laboratory findings from research studies that appear to discriminate between groups in highly selected and artificially enriched research samples should be the focus of subsequent diagnostic research in an attempt to research whether such laboratory findings may have diagnostic value, in terms of a sufficiently elevated likelihood ratio, in routine clinical practice settings. It would be useful to compile a list of diagnostic likelihood ratios of these measures, taking into account the setting and the base prevalence of the disorder to be diagnosed in that particular setting, and use these to develop quantitative diagnostic algorithms and decision trees in a new module in the DSM and ICD systems. This approach is further discussed at the end of this chapter.

TEMPORAL STABILITY OF BIPOLAR DISORDER: ASSESSING PREDICTIVE VALIDITY

Temporal stability may be invoked as a criterion for assessing the validity of psychiatric diagnosis as far as the category in question is supposed to be stable over

TABLE 4–1. Predominant polarity correlates

Depressive polarity	Manic polarity
60% bipolar patients	40% bipolar patients
More bipolar II	More bipolar I
More depressive onset	More manic onset
More seasonal pattern	Younger and earlier onset
More suicide attempts	More substance misuse
Better long-term response to lamotrigine	Better long-term response to atypical antipsychotics
More antidepressant use	

time. Diagnostic reliability may also influence predictive validity, as poor reliability might hamper the theoretical stability of a certain diagnostic category. Follow-up studies are crucial to assess predictive validity. Categories that include chronicity as part of their definition are more likely to be temporally stable (e.g., schizophrenia), whereas others are unstable almost by definition (e.g., schizophreniform disorder). In bipolar disorder, bipolar I is more stable than bipolar II just because bipolar II may switch to bipolar I, but not vice versa. The stability of bipolar disorder has generally been reported to be high, ranging from 70% to 91%.[33–36]

Certain situations that may be developed by patients over time, but that may not be part of the core syndrome but rather a particular longitudinal pattern, are included in current classifications as course specifiers. For bipolar disorder, they include chronicity (with or without full interepisode recovery), seasonality, and rapid cycling. A further potential specifier for DSM-V may be "predominant polarity." As many as 56% of bipolar patients display a specific pattern of predominant polarity; 60% of those may be classified as predominantly depressed (with at least two-thirds of past episodes fulfilling criteria for major depression), whereas 40% may be classified as predominantly manic or hypomanic.[37] Table 4–1 shows the characteristics of the two groups.

A Proposal for DSM-V and ICD-11

OVERCOMING THE CATEGORICAL VERSUS DIMENSIONAL APPROACH DILEMMA

The only way to overcome the problems associated with either the categorical or the dimensional approach is to adopt both. As discussed above, the dimensional approach may be closer to reality but may carry reliability problems and be difficult to implement in real life, including aspects with important financial and social

TABLE 4–2. A proposal for dimensional classification as a further axis or module for the classification of mental disorders

Dimension/severity	None (absent)	Mild	Moderate	Severe
Psychotic (positive) symptoms	0	1	2	3
Negative symptoms	0	1	2	3
Manic symptoms	0	1	2	3
Depressive symptoms	0	1	2	3
Cognitive impairment	0	1	2	3
Anxiety	0	1	2	3
Obsessive-compulsive symptoms	0	1	2	3
Substance misuse	0	1	2	3
Impulsivity	0	1	2	3
Suicidality	0	1	2	3
Eating problems	0	1	2	3
Sleeping problems	0	1	2	3
Sexual problems	0	1	2	3

implications such as reimbursement policies, insurance issues, and drug regulations; on the other hand, the categorical approach has proved to be unsatisfactory with regard to diagnostic validity and has carried problems such as inflated comorbidity rates and a growing number of diagnostic categories (psychiatry is probably the only medical specialty where the number of conditions is continuously increasing rather than decreasing); however, the categorical approach is practical, easy, and reliable. We believe that switching from a categorical to a dimensional classification would be unfeasible and extremely confusing, but we also think that the time has come to include some dimensional information in the system. In this regard, we propose the development of a dimensional module within the categorical classification that may end up to be extremely helpful for research, teaching, and clinical practice, by allowing to assess in a systematic way a limited number of issues, as listed in Table 4–2. These dimensions have been thought to work for the majority of mental disorders, not just bipolar disorder. Patients would eventually be rated according to whether the specific dimension is present with mild, moderate, or severe intensity, or is absent. Of course, every dimension should be very well defined a priori, and high scores in any dimension would deserve further specifications in every case, but this would be a simple way to start to develop a complementary dimensional view over our rigid and poorly valid taxonomy.

TABLE 4–3.　Limitations of current diagnostic criteria for bipolar disorder

- Psychotic symptoms are common in mania and may also happen in depression, but they are not part of the diagnostic criteria, reinforcing the idea that psychosis is a core feature of schizophrenia but not bipolar disorder
- Mood-congruent vs. mood-incongruent psychotic symptoms are not well defined
- Bipolar depression is undistinguishable from unipolar major depression
- Recurring depressions are not recognized as a potential precursor to bipolar disorder—may be diagnosed as a depressive disorder
- Mixed symptoms are not sufficiently characterized, and mixed episodes are too narrowly defined
- Cognitive symptoms are not included
- Drug-induced mania and hypomania are excluded: problems in judging what "direct physiological consequence of a drug, medication, or somatic treatment" means
- No account is taken of family history and biological markers
- Four-day duration required for diagnosis of hypomania and 1 week for mania may be too long
- Bipolar disorder not-otherwise-specified may include the majority of cases, particularly in children and adolescents

---

REFINING CURRENT DIAGNOSTIC CRITERIA

As mentioned, we do not want the categorical classification to disappear. In fact, the dimensional module would be a poor contribution if we were not able to refine, at the same time, the current nosology. Refinements should be data driven. Further research is needed to assess the sensitivity and specificity of diagnostic criteria and categories. Some of the specific problems related to the diagnosis of bipolar disorder and issues that require urgent revision are listed in Table 4–3.

THE MODULAR APPROACH

The modular approach aims to be a step forward for the axial approach, which proved successful in DSM-III but has become partially obsolete. The modular approach includes a first module that basically corresponds to a refined Axis I in current classification but also includes some of the categories included in Axis II, such as certain conditions controversially classified as personality disorders (i.e., borderline disorder); module I is the clinical diagnostic classification in which some hierarchical issues (primary vs. secondary, etc.) may or may not be included. Module

TABLE 4–4.   Proposal for a modular approach to the classification and diagnosis of people with mental disorders

Module I	Categorical classification
Module II	Dimensional assessment
Module III	Laboratory data
Module IV	Medical nonpsychiatric conditions
Module V	Psychological assessment
Module VI	Social issues (environmental factors and social function)

II involves the dimensional approach and includes a limited number of potential symptomatic dimensions (see Table 4–2 for a preliminary proposal), which can be dimensionally rated regardless of the diagnostic category according to module I. Module III is the laboratory module and should include all the items in the psychiatric toolbox (genotypation, structural and functional neuroimaging, REM latency, hormonal tests, cognitive data) that would enhance diagnostic validity. In Chapter 10, we therefore discuss further the extent to which findings from recent structural and functional neuroimaging studies in particular might have increased our ability to identify potential biomarkers of bipolar disorder to indeed enhance the diagnostic validity of the disorder. The modular approach allows for a simple clinical diagnosis when such tools are not available or not cost effective but permits integration of the biological data as well when appropriate and is the first step toward a future classification based on pathophysiological grounds. Module IV corresponds to Axis III in DSM and probably requires further attention, especially for some nonpsychiatric conditions that are overrepresented in the mentally ill and are likely to influence and to be influenced by the psychiatric disorder (e.g., diabetes, obesity, cancer, cardiovascular disease). The medical morbidity in bipolar disorder is extremely high and rapidly increasing.[38] Module V should be the psychological module and should include all the information about personality and usual behavior of the subject that may be relevant for psychiatric assessment. Some, but not all, of the items and categories currently included in DSM's Axis II should go here. This module should necessarily have a dimensional format, avoiding all the problems related to poor validity and reliability of personality disorders as described in DSM-IV and ICD-10. Finally, the social issues should be assessed in module VI, including what is currently included in Axes IV and V of DSM-IV, namely psychosocial and environmental problems and social functioning. A summary of the modular approach is shown in Table 4–4.

In conclusion, the validity of psychiatric diagnosis in general and bipolar disorder in particular deserves further research and alternative approaches. There is a clear need to improve and refine the current diagnostic criteria and to introduce dimensions not as an alternative but rather as a useful complement to categorical diagnosis. Laboratory, family, and treatment response data should also be systematically included in the diagnostic assessment when available. There is little chance that DSM-V or ICD-11 may represent a true step forward if these kinds of data are not included. We propose a modular system that may integrate categorical and dimensional issues, laboratory data, associated nonpsychiatric medical conditions, psychological assessment, and social issues in a comprehensive and nevertheless practical approach.

References

1. Jablensky A. The conflict of the nosologists: views on schizophrenia and manic-depressive illness in the early part of the 20th century. Schizophr Res. 1999;39:95–100.
2. Boteva K, Lieberman J. Reconsidering the classification of schizophrenia and manic depressive illness—a critical analysis and new conceptual model. World J Biol Psychiatry. 2003;4:81–92.
3. American Psychiatric Association. Diagnostic and Statistical Manual of Mental Disorders. 4th ed, Text Revision. Washington, DC: American Psychiatric Association; 2000.
4. World Health Organization. International Statistical Classification of Diseases and Related Health Problems. 10th ed. Geneva, Switzerland: World Health Organization; 1992.
5. Robins E, Guze SB. Establishment of diagnostic validity in psychiatric illness: its application to schizophrenia. Am J Psychiatry. 1970;126:983–987.
6. Feighner JP, Robins E, Guze SB, Woodruff RA Jr, Winokur G, Munoz R. Diagnostic criteria for use in psychiatric research. Arch Gen Psychiatry. 1972;26:57–63.
7. American Psychiatric Association. Diagnostic and Statistical Manual of Mental Disorders. 3rd ed. Washington, DC: American Psychiatric Association; 1980.
8. American Psychiatric Association. Diagnostic and Statistical Manual of Mental Disorders. 3rd ed Revised. Washington, DC: American Psychiatric Association; 1987.
9. American Psychiatric Association. Diagnostic and Statistical Manual of Mental Disorders. 4th ed. Washington, DC: American Psychiatric Association; 1994.
10. Goodwin FK, Jamison KR. Manic-Depressive Illness. New York: Oxford University Press; 1990.
11. Akiskal HS, Bourgeois ML, Angst J, Post R, Moller H, Hirschfeld R. Re-evaluating the prevalence of and diagnostic composition within the broad clinical spectrum of bipolar disorders. J Affect Disord. 2000;59(suppl 1):S5–S30.
12. Suppes T, Mintz J, McElroy SL, et al. Mixed hypomania in 908 patients with bipolar disorder evaluated prospectively in the Stanley Foundation Bipolar Treatment Network: a sex-specific phenomenon. Arch Gen Psychiatry. 2005;62:1089–1096.
13. World Health Organization. International Statistical Classification of Diseases and Related Health Problems. 9th ed. Geneva, Switzerland: World Health Organization; 1977.
14. American Psychiatric Association. Diagnostic and Statistical Manual of Mental Disorders. 2nd ed. Washington, DC: American Psychiatric Association; 1968.
15. Taylor MA, Abrams R, Gaztanaga P. Manic-depressive illness and schizophrenia: a partial validation of research diagnostic criteria utilizing neuropsychological testing. Compr Psychiatry. 1975;16:91–96.

16. Schumacher J, Jamra RA, Freudenberg J, et al. Examination of G72 and D-amino-acid oxidase as genetic risk factors for schizophrenia and bipolar affective disorder. Mol Psychiatry. 2004;9:203–207.
17. Berrettini W. Evidence for shared susceptibility in bipolar disorder and schizophrenia. Am J Med Genet C Semin Med Genet. 2003;123:59–64.
18. Potash JB. Carving chaos: genetics and the classification of mood and psychotic syndromes. Harv Rev Psychiatry. 2006;14:47–63.
19. McDonald C, Bullmore ET, Sham PC, et al. Association of genetic risks for schizophrenia and bipolar disorder with specific and generic brain structural endophenotypes. Arch Gen Psychiatry. 2004;61:974–984.
20. Blumberg HP, Fredericks C, Wang F, et al. Preliminary evidence for persistent abnormalities in amygdala volumes in adolescents and young adults with bipolar disorder. Bipolar Disord. 2005;7:570–576.
21. Benabarre A, Vieta E, Martínez-Arán A, et al. The somatics of psyche: structural neuromorphometry of bipolar disorders. Psychother Psychosom. 2002;71:180–189.
22. Martínez-Arán A, Penades R, Vieta E, et al. Executive function in patients with remitted bipolar disorder and schizophrenia and its relationship with functional outcome. Psychother Psychosom. 2002;71:39–46.
23. Altshuler LL, Ventura J, van Gorp WG, Green MF, Theberge DC, Mintz J. Neurocognitive function in clinically stable men with bipolar I disorder or schizophrenia and normal control subjects. Biol Psychiatry. 2004;56:560–569.
24. Daban C, Martínez-Arán A, Torrent C, et al. Specificity of cognitive deficits in bipolar disorder versus schizophrenia. A systematic review. Psychother Psychosom. 2006;75:72–84.
25. Cannon M, Caspi A, Moffitt TE, et al. Evidence for early childhood, pan-developmental impairment specific to schizophreniform disorder: results from a longitudinal birth cohort. Arch Gen Psychiatry. 2002;59:449–456.
26. Reichenberg A, Weiser M, Rabinowitz J, et al. A population-based cohort study of premorbid intellectual, language, and behavioral functioning in patients with schizophrenia, schizoaffective disorder, and nonpsychotic bipolar disorder. Am J Psychiatry. 2002;159:2027–2035.
27. Zammit S, Allebeck P, David AS, et al. A longitudinal study of premorbid IQ score and risk of developing schizophrenia, bipolar disorder, severe depression, and other nonaffective psychoses. Arch Gen Psychiatry. 2004;61:354–360.
28. Leucht S, Kissling W, McGrath J. Lithium for schizophrenia revisited: a systematic review and meta-analysis of randomized controlled trials. J Clin Psychiatry. 2004;65:177–186.
29. Goodwin FK, Murphy DL, Dunner DL, Bunney WE Jr. Lithium response in unipolar versus bipolar depression. Am J Psychiatry. 1972;129:44–47.
30. Vieta E. The role of third-generation anticonvulsants in the treatment of bipolar disorder. Clin Neuropsychiatry. 2004;1:159–164.
31. Grof P, Duffy A, Cavazzoni P, et al. Is response to prophylactic lithium a familial trait? J Clin Psychiatry. 2002;63:942–947.
32. Peet M. Induction of mania with selective serotonin re-uptake inhibitors and tricyclic antidepressants. Br J Psychiatry. 1994;164:549–550.

33. Amin S, Singh SP, Brewin J, Jones PB, Medley I, Harrison G. Diagnostic stability of first-episode psychosis. Comparison of ICD-10 and DSM-III-R systems. Br J Psychiatry. 1999;175:537–543.

34. Schwartz JE, Fennig S, Tanenberg-Karant M, et al. Congruence of diagnoses 2 years after a first-admission diagnosis of psychosis. Arch Gen Psychiatry. 2000;57:593–600.

35. Schimmelmann BG, Conus P, Edwards J, McGorry PD, Lambert M. Diagnostic stability 18 months after treatment initiation for first-episode psychosis. J Clin Psychiatry. 2005;66:1239–1246.

36. Kessing LV. Diagnostic stability in bipolar disorder in clinical practise as according to ICD-10. J Affect Disord. 2005;85:293–299.

37. Colom F, Vieta E, Daban C, Pacchiarotti I, Sanchez-Moreno J. Clinical and therapeutic implications of predominant polarity in bipolar disorder. J Affect Disord. 2006;93:13–17.

38. Kupfer DJ. The increasing medical burden in bipolar disorder. JAMA. 2005;293:2528–2530.

5

DSM-V RESEARCH AGENDA

Substance Abuse/Psychosis Comorbidity

Bruce J. Rounsaville, M.D.

DSM-V Research Agenda:
Substance Abuse/Psychosis Comorbidity

One of the most common challenges for psychiatric diagnosis is posed by patients who experience the onset of psychotic symptoms during episodes of current or recent psychoactive substance use.[1] In *Diagnostic and Statistical Manual of Mental Disorders,* 4th Edition (DSM-IV),[2] all major categories of nonorganic psychotic disorders include an exclusion criterion that "symptoms are not *due to* the direct physiological effects of a substance" (e.g., p. 327, Major Depressive Episode, emphasis added). In practice, determining whether a given psychotic symptom is "due to" drug effects is far from straightforward. In a study of first episodes of psychosis, Fennig and colleagues[3] were unable to make a clear diagnosis in 25/278 cases, and substance abuse was the most common cause of diagnostic ambiguity. Shaner and colleagues[4] characterized the sources of diagnostic confusion in a study

Reprinted with permission from Rounsaville BJ. "DSM-V Research Agenda: Substance Abuse/Psychosis Comorbidity." *Schizophrenia Bulletin* 2007; 33: 947–952.

This work was supported in part by grants K05 DA00089 and P50DA09241 from the National Institute on Drug Abuse and the U.S. Veterans Administration New England Mental Illness Research, Education, and Clinical Center.

of 165 patients with chronic psychosis and substance abuse on whom a "definitive diagnosis" could not be arrived at. Most common factors clouding diagnosis were identified as insufficient abstinence (78%), poor memory (24%), and inconsistent reporting (20%). While current substance abuse in psychotic patients poses practical challenges for the diagnostic *process,* do these diagnostic dilemmas point to the need for changes in the DSM-IV diagnostic *criteria?* In this chapter, I will review DSM-IV guidelines for diagnosing comorbid psychotic disorders and substance use disorders (SUDs), the factors undermining definitive diagnosis of comorbid disorders, potential nosological changes that could address these issues, and the types of research that could inform a revision of criteria and guidelines for diagnosing comorbid SUDs and psychosis.

DSM-IV Guidelines for Diagnosing Comorbid Psychotic Disorders and SUDs

In keeping with the atheoretical and phenomenological principles of St. Louis psychiatry,[5,6] DSM-IV encourages listing all diagnoses, past and present, for which a patient meets criteria. For patients with SUDs, psychotic disorders can be diagnosed as "independent" or subsumed under one of the many "substance-induced" mental disorders of which psychosis is a feature. With variations related to the pharmacological effects of different categories of substances (e.g., alcohol, opioids, stimulants), these include acute intoxication, intoxication delirium, withdrawal, alcohol-induced persistent dementia, and substance-induced psychotic disorder with hallucinations. Because "independent" psychotic diagnoses (e.g., schizophrenia, bipolar I) are not to be made if symptoms are due to effects of substances, newly emerging psychotic symptoms in the presence of substance abuse (or withdrawal) are presumed to be "substance induced" until proven otherwise. In psychotic patients who use substances, evidence for "independence" of psychotic symptoms requires onset of symptoms during a drug-free period or persistence of psychotic symptoms during a period of sustained abstinence from psychoactive substances (when intoxication or withdrawal effects can no longer account for psychotic symptoms). Except for alcohol-induced pathological dementia, all the substance-induced psychotic mental disorders are considered to be time limited.

Difficulties in Applying DSM-IV Guidelines for Diagnosing Comorbid SUDs and Psychotic Disorders

Disentangling the relationship between SUDs and psychotic disorders is a commonplace diagnostic challenge both for clinicians in treatment settings and for researchers in community settings. U.S. community surveys, such as the Epidemiology Catchment Area and National Comorbidity Survey, document an association of most classes of mental disorders with SUDs, with a particularly high association between bipolar disorder and SUDs.[7,8] Clinical samples of patients with schizophrenia and bipolar disorder report even higher rates of SUDs, suggesting that comorbidity contributes to treatment seeking.[9–12] In fact, for patients with both comorbid SUDs and schizophrenia, rehospitalization is frequently associated with relapse to drug use along with discontinuation of prescribed antipsychotic medications.[10,12]

When patients present with current or recent substance abuse and psychosis, the key diagnostic question is whether or not the psychotic symptoms are accounted for by the substance use. If so, then antipsychotic treatment can be seen as short term while central emphasis is placed on substance abuse treatment. If not, then major emphasis must be placed on long-term care of the independent psychotic disorder, as these disorders tend to be chronic and associated with severe and sustained psychosocial impairment.[1] Psychotic syndromes can be considered as "independent" of substance use if they have an age of onset prior to the onset of SUDs or if psychotic and other symptoms persist during sustained drug-free periods. Another central differential diagnostic feature of "independent" psychotic disorders is that they are characterized by having a clear sensorium, as disorientation is a key feature of the delirium that is associated with many substance-induced psychotic syndromes. In practice, several features of comorbid SUDs and psychosis cloud the picture. First, patients may report no sustained drug-free periods. Both SUDs and psychotic disorders are chronic conditions that most typically begin during teen years or young adulthood. Once a pattern of sustained drug abuse begins, sustained periods of abstinence may be absent or infrequent. If psychotic symptoms emerge during periods of heavy drug use, these may indeed be "substance induced," but they may also be manifestations of an independent illness that happens to be emerging at the same time or that may be precipitated by the concurrent substance use. Second, it is difficult to establish or practice precise guidelines for specifying the amount of time that defines a "sustained drug-free period." For hospitalized or closely supervised patients, treatment may lead to detoxification from substances, but lengthy inpatient stays are now the exception and not the rule. Moreover, substance-induced psychotic symptoms may persist long after cessation of use. For example, a recent review of studies of stimulant-induced psychoses noted that 1%–15% of patients had psychotic symptoms that persisted greater than 1 month.[13] Further complications arise for patients who abuse multiple substances, each with a differing profile of psychotogenic effects and duration of withdrawal syndromes. Third, patients with comorbid psychotic disorders and substance abuse are likely to have a poor memory of the precise sequence of events that occurred during their teens, such as pinpointing the onset of initial psychotic symptoms versus the initiation of heavy substance use. Fourth, establishment of a "clear sensorium" is difficult even in acutely psychotic patients who do not use substances because of cognitive deficits, confusion, and difficulty in cooperating with the examiner. Fifth, the profile of psychotic symptoms associated with heavy substance use (particularly of stimulants) is difficult to distinguish from independent psychotic disorders. For example, a recent review of stimulant-induced psychosis[13] documented the following rates of reported symptoms: paranoia (25%–75%), auditory hallucinations (50%–80%), ideas of references (15%–60%), Schneiderian first-rank symptoms (up to 50%), and negative symptoms (5%–30%).

Emerging Findings on Substance-Induced Psychotic Disorders

In addition to the everyday practical challenges to differentiating "substance-induced" from "independent" psychotic disorders, a major issue related to the etiology of psychotic disorders is whether or not psychoactive substance use can be considered a "cause" of schizophrenia, a condition that has been traditionally thought of as "independent" of substance use. Recent interest has focused on the relationship of teen and young adult cannabis use to increased risk for a subsequent diagnosis of schizophrenia. In a meta-analytic review of seven longitudinal studies, Henquet and colleagues[14] reported a 2.1 odds ratio for increased risk for schizophrenia in cannabis users. Intriguing clues for a possible genetic basis for this increased use have been reported by Caspi and colleagues[15] who documented a stronger association between cannabis use and schizophrenia for subjects with the Val-Val variant of the *COMT* gene. From a nosological standpoint, research of this type raises important questions about the definition of the schizophrenia syndrome itself. Are episodes of "schizophrenia" that are induced by cannabis use identical with those that are not? If not, then some type of designation of a subgroup of schizophrenia would be useful for denoting this substance-induced variant. Alternatively, if the cannabis-induced syndromes are identical to independent syndromes, this suggests the value of studying cannabis effects to identify neurobiological processes underlying schizophrenia. As noted above, aside from alcohol-induced dementia, substance-induced psychoses have traditionally been considered to be time limited, and the role of drugs in causing more enduring psychoses has been that of precipitating or facilitating expression of an underlying psychotic process.

How Can DSM-V Address Diagnostic Challenges and Emerging Findings?

In considering the potential nosological impact of emerging findings about substance-induced psychotic disorder or difficulties in distinguishing "substance-induced" from "independent" psychoses, it is important to recall that clinical challenges in diagnosis or new etiological findings have no straightforward relationship to amending the diagnostic system itself. The difficulties in distinguishing substance-induced from independent psychotic symptoms are hardly new and were well known to framers of DSM-III,[16] DSM-III-R,[17] and DSM-IV criteria. The current guidelines embody the thinking of previous work groups on the optimal way of handling these issues. Likewise, the impact of drug use on etiology of schizophrenia is one of many factors contributing to the disorder, and the general policy of the DSM and ICD *(International Classification of Diseases)* systems is to base diagnostic groupings on phenomenology of disorders and not on causes, given the lack of definitive knowledge about causes of any of the major mental disorders.[18]

If changes are to be made in DSM-IV related to comorbid psychotic disorders and SUDs, these can take place at several different levels including a) rearrangement of groups of disorders (e.g., subsuming SUDs, eating disorders, and impulse control disorders under a general category of "Addictions" or "Impulse Control Disorders"); b) adding or deleting a diagnostic category; c) changing diagnostic criteria; or d) changing textual guidelines for determining the presence or absence of criteria. Response to the problems of differentiating substance-induced versus independent disorders would most likely be in the text or in the criteria for specific substance-induced syndromes. Changes made on the basis of emerging findings about enduring psychoses caused by drug abuse could be at the syndrome level (e.g., adding a "cannabis-induced enduring psychosis" diagnosis) or in the text describing characteristics of disorders.

To inform the diagnostic decision between substance-induced and independent psychotic symptoms, two kinds of information would be useful: 1) identification of early markers that clearly differentiate the two conditions and 2) more precise information about the duration of substance-induced psychotic symptoms. At present, the most definitive method for making this distinction is longitudinal assessment after a period of sustained abstinence from psychoactive substances. This is time consuming and often impractical given the relapsing nature of substance abuse and limited access to inpatient care. First, more rapid diagnosis could be facilitated by the identification of "markers" or distinctive clinical features that would identify patients with psychotic symptoms as having transient, substance-induced syndromes or enduring independent disorders. Such markers might take the form of biological indices (e.g., a genetic profile suggesting schizophrenia), symptom profiles, or features of the psychiatric history. Recent work by Caton and colleagues[19] and unpublished data by C.L.M. Caton, D.S. Hasin, P.E. Shrout, R.E. Drake, B. Bominguez, S. Samet, and B. Shanzer illustrate this approach. In a sample of 319 treatment-entering patients with psychosis and SUDs, reevaluation at 1-year follow-up revealed that 25% of psychotic diagnoses that had originally been designated as substance-induced were reclassified as independent. At initial evaluation, the reclassified patients differed from those with transient psychoses by being more likely to report parental mental illness, having poorer pre-morbid adjustment, and having less insight into their psychosis. Second, more definitive information could be gathered on the duration of substance-induced psychotic symptoms and syndromes. Numerous studies have evaluated characteristics and course of stimulant-induced psychosis,[13,20–23] but less is known about the time course of transient psychotic syndromes resulting from use of other classes of drugs or from polysubstance abuse. At present, for purposes of differential diagnosis, "sustained" remission is considered to be around 4 weeks of abstinence. Conceivably, this duration of abstinence may be too short for psychoses induced by some substances (e.g., cannabis or hallucinogens) or too long for those induced by others (e.g., benzodiazepines).

Recent evidence suggesting that cannabis use may contribute as a cause of "schizophrenia" diagnosis[14] could have an important impact on the understanding of psychotic illnesses and on the system for classifying these illnesses. From a practical, clinical standpoint, intervening with teenage marijuana use could prevent the development of a full psychotic syndrome in susceptible individuals. Such a preventive substance abuse intervention could be coupled with early antipsychotic pharmacotherapy to intervene in the "prodromal" period of schizophrenia or other psychotic conditions.[24] For understanding etiology, research on mechanisms of cannabis effects may point to neurobiological pathways underlying vulnerability to schizophrenia. Nosological changes that might be made on the basis of these findings would require considerably more evidence than is currently available. For example, enduring psychotic syndromes associated with prior cannabis use may constitute disorders that are distinctly different from what is now called "schizophrenia" and that would warrant classification as separate disorders. Delineation of such a syndrome (or syndromes) would require a considerable body of work documenting diagnostic distinctiveness, course, symptom features, and other types of evidence articulated by Robins and Guze[5] for defining psychiatric disorders. Alternatively, the concept of schizophrenia that is "caused" by cannabis use suggests the possibility of designating subtypes of psychotic disorders on the basis of differing etiological factors, which could include genetic, developmental, or other causes.

Adding Substance Use to the Research Agenda on Nosology of Psychosis

Heterogeneity within categories of psychotic disorders (e.g., schizophrenia) and lack of clear boundaries between major subtypes (e.g., mood-related psychoses and schizophrenia) are major challenges for current official nomenclatures for psychotic disorders. These two general problems run through most of the papers in this series.[25] An additional challenge for defining homogenous, distinctive subtypes based on etiology and pathophysiology is posed by highly prevalent comorbid abuse and dependence on psychoactive substances that can cause at least temporary psychotic symptoms. For example, use of stimulants by schizophrenic patients may cause euphoria after initial use followed by a dysphoric "crash" that may mimic bipolar disorder.[9] Alternatively, use of stimulants by schizophrenic patients may, in itself, be an indicator of manic disinhibition and point to a diagnosis of schizoaffective disorder.

An improved diagnostic system for comorbid psychotic disorders and SUDs must arise from a better understanding of the relationship between these two broad classes of disorders. Research to clarify these relationships could be most efficiently conducted by two general strategies: 1) reanalysis of longitudinal surveys that include diagnoses of SUDs and psychotic disorder and 2) including patients with comorbid disorders in studies of the neurobiology and/or treatment of psychotic disorders.

As a first general strategy, important clues about the relationship between SUDs and psychoses can be gained through reanalysis of existing longitudinal data sets of community and clinical samples. Robins[26] has recently advocated this approach for addressing nomenclature issues generally and identifies several major studies with longitudinal components, including the Epidemiologic Catchment Area Study,[27] the National Comorbidity Survey,[28] and the Detroit studies of Breslau and colleagues.[29] A more comprehensive review of public access data from community surveys of SUDs is provided by Cottler and Grant.[30] Issues that could be addressed in these analyses include the relationship of SUDs diagnosed in early waves to the onset of new psychotic disorders diagnosed at later waves or the relationship of SUDs to diagnostic instability of psychotic disorders across waves. For example, secondary analysis of data from existing longitudinal studies was the approach used for many of the reports on cannabis and increased risk for schizophrenic disorders reviewed by Henquet et al.[14]

A second general strategy to improve understanding of the SUD/psychosis relationship would be to include subjects with comorbid disorders in the full range of research projects for which the goal is to elucidate the etiology, pathophysiology, and treatment of psychotic disorders. Despite the high rates of psychoactive substance use in clinical populations of psychotic patients, research on the treatment and neurobiology of psychotic disorders tends to avoid potential confounds by excluding psychotic subjects with current substance abuse. Excluding substance-abusing patients from, for example, neuroimaging studies of bipolar patients has considerable merit for eliminating drug effects that might be mistakenly attributed to the bipolar disorder itself. However, findings from such research may not be generalized to bipolar patients who abuse substances and whose conditions could represent a distinct diagnostic subtype. In addition to scientific barriers to study of psychotic patients with comorbid SUDs, the organization of U.S. National Institutes of Health research support creates another barrier to this type of research.

Most research on psychoses is supported by the National Institute of Mental Health, whereas research on SUDs is supported by separate institutes (i.e., the National Institute on Drug Abuse and the National Institute on Alcoholism and Alcohol Abuse). While conjoint support across institutes is a possibility, such an arrangement is not the norm.

A third general strategy to elucidate the relationship between SUDs and psychotic disorders would be to initiate descriptive phenomenological studies that capture the onset of SUDs and nonorganic psychotic disorders. Informative samples for this research could include high risk, psychotic family history, positive teens and young adults who exhibit prodromal psychotic symptoms,[24] or patients seeking treatment for a first episode of psychosis.[3]

DSM-V and Beyond

In reviewing literature on comorbid psychosis and SUDs coming out after publication of DSM-IV, I was unable to locate published criticism of those aspects of the official nomenclature that specifically address the intersection between psychotic disorders and SUDs. This relative absence of discontent strongly contrasts with criticisms embodied in other papers in this series[25] pointing out the lack of clear boundaries between psychotic diagnoses related to mood disorders versus nonaffective psychoses, the unacceptably large heterogeneity within diagnostic subgroups, and the limitations of a categorical approach to the diagnosis of psychotic disorders. Ultimately, the ideal psychiatric nomenclature will define syndromes on the basis of established etiology and/or pathophysiology. For patients with comorbid psychosis and SUDs, this association may be explained by chance, shared common etiological factors for the two disorders, substance use contributing to the etiology of psychosis, or psychosis contributing to the etiology of SUDs. At present, except for the relatively narrow and transient group of "substance-induced" psychoses, the current diagnostic system is silent about hierarchical or causal relationships between disorders when patients qualify for multiple diagnoses. With emerging advances in knowledge about the shared etiology and neurobiology of SUDs and psychoses, these relationships may be reflected in a more advanced nomenclature. Looking toward DSM-V, no emerging findings related to either type of disorder can be said to justify major changes in the ways that psychosis/SUD comorbidity is currently diagnosed. In the absence of compelling need and a strong empirical basis for change, diagnostic conservatism is called for. It is important to remember the many costs of enacting major changes in nosology and to set a relatively high threshold for revision. These costs include the burden on clinicians, who must learn a new system; disruptions in research, particularly in longitudinal studies and in the ability to compare past and future studies; apparent changes in prevalence rates, which mainly reflect artifacts of syndrome definitions; the need to modify existing instruments or develop new instruments; and a negative public perception of vacillation or uncertainty.[6,31]

References

1. Rosenthal RN, Miner CR. Differential diagnosis of substance-induced psychosis and schizophrenia in patients with substance use disorders. Schizophr Bull. 1997;23:187–193.
2. American Psychiatric Association. Diagnostic and Statistical Manual of Mental Disorders. 4th ed. Washington, DC: American Psychiatric Association; 1994.
3. Fennig S, Bromet EJ, Craig T, Jandorf L, Schwartz JE. Psychotic patients with unclear diagnoses: a descriptive analysis. J Nerv Ment Dis. 1995;183:207–213.
4. Shaner A, Roberts LJ, Racenstein JM, Eckman TA, Tsuang JW, Tucker DE. Sources of diagnostic uncertainty among chronically psychotic cocaine abusers. 149th Annual Meeting of the American Psychiatric Association; May 4–9, 1996; New York.
5. Robins E, Guze SB. Establishment of diagnostic validity in psychiatric illness: its application to schizophrenia. Am J Psychiatry. 1970;126:983–987.
6. Kendler KS. Toward a scientific psychiatric nosology: strengths and limitations. Arch Gen Psychiatry. 1990;47:969–973.
7. Kessler RC, Crum RM, Warner LA, Nelson CB, Schulenberg J, Anthony JC. Lifetime co-occurrence of DSM-III-R alcohol abuse and dependence with other psychiatric disorders in the National Comorbidity Survey. Arch Gen Psychiatry. 1997;54:313–321.
8. Regier DA, Farmer ME, Rae DS, et al. Comorbidity of mental disorders with alcohol and other drug abuse: results from the Epidemiological Catchment Area (ECA) Study. JAMA. 1990;264:2511–2518.
9. Ziedonis D, Steinberg ML, D'Avanzo K, Smelson D. Co-occurring schizophrenia and addiction. In: Kranzler HR, Tinsley JA, eds. Dual Diagnosis and Psychiatric Treatment: Substance Abuse and Comorbid Disorders. 2nd ed. New York: Marcel Dekker; 1998:427–466.
10. Mueser KT, Bellack AS, Blanchard JJ. Comorbidity of schizophrenia and substance abuse: implications for treatment. J Consult Clin Psychol. 1992;47:1102–1114.
11. Lehman AF, Myers CP, Corty E, Thompson JW. Prevalence and patterns of "dual diagnosis" among psychiatric inpatients. Compr Psychiatry. 1994;35:106–112.
12. Schneier FR, Siris SG. A review of psychoactive substance use and abuse in schizophrenia. Patterns of drug choice. J Nerv Ment Dis. 1987;175:641–652.
13. Schuckit MA. Comorbidity between substance use disorders and psychiatry conditions. Addiction. 2006;101(suppl 1):76–88.
14. Henquet C, Murray R, Linszen D, van Os J. The environment and schizophrenia: the role of cannabis use. Schizophr Bull. 2005;31:608–612.
15. Caspi A, Moffitt TE, Cannon M, et al. Moderation of the effect of adolescent-onset cannabis use on adult psychosis by a functional polymorphism in the catechol-*O*-methyltransferase gene: longitudinal evidence of a gene x environment interaction. Biol Psychiatry. 2005;57:1117–1127.

16. American Psychiatric Association. Diagnostic and Statistical Manual of Mental Disorders. 3rd ed. Washington, DC: American Psychiatric Association; 1980.

17. American Psychiatric Association. Diagnostic and Statistical Manual of Mental Disorders. 3rd ed Revised. Washington, DC: American Psychiatric Association; 1987.

18. Kendall RE. The distinction between mental and physical illness. Br J Psychiatry. 2001;178:490–493.

19. Caton CLM, Drake RE, Hasin DS, et al. Differences between early phase primary psychotic disorders with concurrent substance use and substance-induced psychosis. Arch Gen Psychiatry. 2005;62:137–145.

20. Chen C-K, Lin S-K, Sham PC, et al. Pre-morbid characteristics and co-morbidity of methamphetamine users with and without psychosis. Psychol Med. 2003;33:1407–1414.

21. Griffith JD. Experimental psychosis induced by the administration of d-amphetamine. In: Costa E, Garattini S, eds. Amphetamine and Related Compounds. New York: Raven Press; 1970:876–904.

22. Janowsky DS, Risch C. Amphetamine psychosis and psychotic symptoms. Psychopharmacology. 1979;65:73–77.

23. Boutros N, Bowers M. Chronic substance-induced psychotic disorders: state of the literature. J Neuropsychiatry Clin Neurosci. 1996;8:470–484.

24. Lee C, McGlashan TH, Wood SW. Prevention of schizophrenia: can it be achieved? CNS Drugs. 2005;19:193–206.

25. van Os J, Tamminga C. Deconstructing psychosis: introduction and overview of special issue. Schizophr Bull. 2007;33:861–862.

26. Robins LN. Using survey results to improve the validity of the standard psychiatric nomenclature. Arch Gen Psychiatry. 2004;61:1188–1194.

27. Swart K, Pratt LA, Armenian HK, Lee LC, Eaton WW. Mental disorders and the incidence of migraine headaches in a community sample: results from the Baltimore Epidemiologic Catchment Area follow-up study. Arch Gen Psychiatry. 2000;57:945–950.

28. Kessler RC, Berglund P, Demier O, et al. The epidemiology of major depressive disorder, results from the National Comorbidity Survey Replication (NCS-R). JAMA. 2003;289:3095–3105.

29. Breslau N, Peterson ES, Schultz LR, Chilcoat HD, Andreski P. Major depression and stages of smoking: a longitudinal investigation. Arch Gen Psychiatry. 1998;55:161–166.

30. Cottler LB, Grant BF. Characteristics of nosologically informative data sets that address key diagnostic issues facing the Diagnostic and Statistical Manual of Mental Disorders, fifth edition (DSM-V) and the International Classification of Diseases, eleventh edition (ICD-11) substance use disorders workgroups. Addiction. 2006;101(suppl 1):161–169.

31. Rounsaville BJ, Alarcon RD, Andrews G, Jackson JS, Kendall RE, Kendler K. Basic nomenclature issues. In: Kupfer D, First M, Regier D, eds. APA Research Agenda for DSM-V. Washington, DC: American Psychiatric Association Press; 2002:1–30.

6

THE GENETIC DECONSTRUCTION OF PSYCHOSIS

Michael J. Owen, Ph.D., FRCPsych, FMedSci
Nick Craddock, Ph.D., FRCPsych
Assen Jablensky, M.D., D.M.S.C., FRCPsych, FRANZCP

The majority of genetic studies into the psychoses over the past two decades have been predicated on the double assumption that a) schizophrenia and bipolar disorder, as defined in *Diagnostic and Statistical Manual of Mental Disorders,* 4th Edition (DSM-IV),[1] and *International Classification of Diseases,* 10th Revision,[2] are discrete, "natural" disease entities with distinct etiology and pathogenesis; and b) these disease entities can be identified by current operational diagnostic conventions, which are based on reported subjective symptoms and, to a lesser extent, on deteriorating performance of expected social roles. Data from genetic epidemiology have been called upon to justify the validity of this approach, often referred to as the "Kraepelinian dichotomy."

Reprinted with permission from Owen MJ, Craddock N, Jablensky A. "The Genetic Deconstruction of Psychosis." *Schizophrenia Bulletin* 2007; 33: 905–911.

Owen's and Craddock's work on the genetics of psychosis and mood disorders is funded through grants from the Wellcome Trust and the Medical Research Council. Jablensky's work on the genetics of cognitive deficit in schizophrenia is funded by the National Health and Medical Research Council of Australia. The authors are indebted to all the participants in our studies.

It is important to note that this widely held notion is incorrect. Kraepelin's seminal work, which aggregated three previously described syndromes—hebephrenia, catatonia, and paranoid dementia—into the clinical entity of *dementia praecox* and delimited the latter from manic-depressive insanity, paranoia, and late paraphrenia, introduced order in the previously chaotic field of nosology and laid down the foundation for the current classifications of psychotic disorders. It is not widely known that, in contrast to the narrowly defined manic-depressive psychosis, Kraepelin's dementia praecox was a broad clinical grouping, consisting of nine clinical "forms," also including what today would be termed *schizoaffective disorder* and *mood-incongruent affective psychoses.* However, in 1920, he wrote that "we cannot distinguish satisfactorily between these two illnesses and this brings home the suspicion that our formulation of the problem may be incorrect…the affective and schizophrenic forms of mental disorder do not represent the expression of particular pathological processes, but rather indicate the areas of our personality in which these processes unfold."[3]

Thus, in his later years, Kraepelin continued to develop and refine his ideas about psychiatric diagnoses, and his thinking had in many ways moved on from the dichotomous classification by the end of his life. However, it is not the goal of this chapter to consider Kraepelin's views in relation to modern nosological practice. A discussion of this sort, although of historical interest, is not of direct relevance. Unfortunately, the dichotomous, categorical view of the psychoses was reified in the *Diagnostic and Statistical Manual of Mental Disorders,* 3rd Edition,[4] formulation (and its consequent versions), and most of the genetic, and other, research into psychoses has been based solely on the "given" diagnostic categories of schizophrenia and bipolar disorder as the phenotypes, notwithstanding the fact that their validity has been challenged by emerging data from many fields of psychiatric research.[5–7]

In this chapter, we will first review the key pieces of evidence from genetic epidemiology that there is in fact a genetic overlap between the psychopathological entities that we currently refer to as *bipolar disorder* and *schizophrenia.* We will then review emerging evidence that the two diagnostic categories share specific susceptibility genes and that particular risk alleles may be associated with specific aspects of the phenotype.

Genetic Epidemiology

FAMILY STUDIES

The great majority of family studies have shown increased risks for schizophrenia, schizoaffective disorder, and schizotypal personality disorder in the relatives of probands with schizophrenia.[8] Family studies of bipolar disorder, on the other hand, have shown increased familial risks of bipolar disorder, schizoaffective disorder, and unipolar depression.[9] In contrast, the majority of studies have failed to find a familial relationship between schizophrenia and bipolar disorder.[10–15] Thus, the weight of evidence has traditionally been interpreted to support the view that schizophrenia and bipolar disorder largely breed true.

This conclusion has been challenged by family studies suggesting shared familial risk[16,17] and by the observation that families exist in which some relatives have schizophrenia, some have bipolar disorder, and some have both psychosis and mood disorder.[18] Moreover, the position of schizoaffective disorder has appeared somewhat anomalous in the context of a strict dichotomous view. Thus, schizoaffective disorder occurs at similarly increased rates both in families of probands with schizophrenia[19] and in those of probands with bipolar disorder.[20] Moreover, both schizophrenia and bipolar disorder have been shown to occur at increased rates in families of probands with schizoaffective disorder.[20] This is supported by one of the largest family studies to date, which used the Swedish inpatient case register and obtained data on over 13,000 cases of schizophrenia and 5,000 cases of bipolar disorder.[21] The cross-disorder incidence ratios were robustly increased in siblings and half-siblings for both schizophrenia and bipolar disorder.

TWIN STUDIES

Twin studies tend to be relatively small, given the difficulty in recruiting cases, and related arguments concerning their power can be made. In fact, the early, canonical twin study of Slater and Shields[22] found that nearly as many of the co-twins of schizophrenic probands had affective disorder as had schizophrenia and that there were actually more parents with affective disorder than with schizophrenia. However, this, like other departures from the Kraepelinian model, was attributed to misdiagnosis.[23] There have been few subsequent attempts to explore or challenge diagnostic boundaries using twin studies. An exception was the study by Farmer et al.,[24] who showed in a study of the first half of the Maudsley twin series that affective disorders, particularly those with mood-incongruent psychotic features, are genetically related to schizophrenia.

More recently, Cardno et al.[25] reasoned that overlap in genetic risk factors between schizophrenia and bipolar disorder might have been obscured in twin studies of psychosis because of the adoption of a hierarchical rule that requires that each individual be given a single lifetime diagnosis. Because schizophrenia was placed higher in terms of severity and "organicity," schizophrenic symptoms tended to "trump" those of mood disorder. When Cardno et al.[25] defined syndromes nonhierarchically, they demonstrated a clear overlap in genetic liability between syndromically defined mania and schizophrenia. Their model fitting suggested that whereas some susceptibility genes are specific to schizophrenia and some to bipolar disorder, there is a third group of genes influencing across-the-board susceptibility to schizoaffective disorder, schizophrenia, and bipolar disorder. A graphic illustration of the varied expression of the same set of susceptibility genes is provided by the Maudsley triplets—a set of genetically identical triplets, two of whom had a lifetime diagnosis of schizophrenia and the third a lifetime diagnosis of bipolar disorder.[26]

Molecular Genetic Studies

Most molecular genetic studies of schizophrenia and bipolar disorder have been based upon the assumption that these constitute two independent disorders, with individual studies typically focusing on only one or the other disorder. Cases with a mix of mood and psychotic features, while common, have tended to be ignored or subsumed into some broader category of either schizophrenia or bipolar disorder.

LINKAGE STUDIES

Individual genetic linkage studies and meta-analyses have identified some chromosomal regions for which there is evidence of linkage in both schizophrenia and bipolar disorder. These include regions of 13q, 22q, 18,[27,28] and 6q.[29] The chromosomal regions implicated are wide and contain many genes, so it is not certain that the apparent overlaps reflect the existence of shared genes between the two disorders. We should also remember that it remains possible that any given linkage might be a false positive in at least one of the disorders.

However, the hypothesis that loci exist that influence susceptibility across the schizophrenia-bipolar divide has recently received further support from a genome-wide linkage scan using families selected on the basis of a member with DSM-IV schizoaffective disorder, bipolar type. This study demonstrated genome-wide significant linkage at 1q42 and suggestive linkage at 22q11, with evidence for linkage being contributed equally by "schizophrenia" families (i.e., those where other members had predominantly schizophrenia) and "bipolar" families (i.e., those where other members had predominantly bipolar disorder).[30] It is of interest that two genes that have been implicated in schizophrenia, *DISC1* and catechol-*O*-methyltransferase *(COMT)*, map to 1q42 and 22q11, respectively, and this raises the question of whether either or both of these genes predispose to illness across the schizophrenia-bipolar divide. There is evidence to support this for both *COMT*[31] and *DISC1* (see below).

STUDIES OF INDIVIDUAL GENES

Linkage studies can provide at best indirect evidence for shared genetic effects. More direct evidence has come from reports implicating variation in the same genes as influencing susceptibility to both schizophrenia and bipolar disorder. In most cases, the gene was first implicated in studies of schizophrenia, and the evidence in most cases is strongest for this phenotype. This could reflect the true contribution to the phenotype or may simply reflect the fact that substantially greater resources and samples have been used to date on studies of schizophrenia. We will consider the evidence for each gene in turn.

NRG1

NRG1 was first implicated in schizophrenia in the Icelandic population after a systematic study of 8p21–22 revealed association between schizophrenia and a multimarker haplotype at the 5' end of *NRG1*.[32] Strong evidence for association with the same haplotype, known as HAP_{ICE}, was subsequently found in a large sample from Scotland,[33] with further support coming from our own United Kingdom sample.[34] These and subsequent studies of *NRG1* in schizophrenia have been reviewed recently.[35] Overall, there is strong evidence from several studies that genetic variation in *NRG1* confers risk to schizophrenia, but not all studies have found the same haplotype to be associated and, as yet, specific susceptibility and protective variants have not been identified. *NRG1* has not yet been extensively studied in bipolar disorder. However, in the only published study to date, we found significant evidence for association of HAP_{ICE} with susceptibility to bipolar disorder of a similar magnitude to that seen by us in schizophrenia (odds ratio [OR] = 1.3).[36] In the bipolar cases with predominantly mood-incongruent psychotic features, the effect was greater (OR = 1.7), as was the case in the subset of schizophrenia patients who had experienced mania (OR = 1.6). Pending replication, these findings should be treated with caution, but they suggest that *NRG1* plays a role in influencing susceptibility to both bipolar disorder and schizophrenia and that it may exert a specific effect in the subset of functional psychoses characterized by both manic and mood-incongruent psychotic features.

Dysbindin

Evidence implicating dystrobrevin-binding protein 1 *(DTNBP1)*, also known as dysbindin, in schizophrenia was first reported by Straub et al.,[37] and there is now quite impressive support from a number of studies reviewed recently.[38] However, once again various markers and haplotypes have been associated, and the actual susceptibility variants have yet to be identified. Raybould and colleagues[39] reported the first study of single-nucleotide polymorphisms (SNPs) from dysbindin in bipolar disorder. They found no significant associations in bipolar disorder as a whole but found modestly significant evidence for association in a subset of bipolar cases with predominantly psychotic episodes. This finding suggests that variation in dysbindin confers risk to some aspect of the psychotic syndrome rather than to the DSM-IV schizophrenia phenotype per se, although replication is required. More recently, Breen et al.[40] reported evidence for association with dysbin-din SNPs in a small sample of bipolar patients, though no analyses stratified by phenotype were conducted. Recent work in the Irish Study of High-Density Schizophrenia Families has shown that schizophrenic patients with negative symptoms were more likely to inherit the dysbindin risk haplotype,[41] raising the possibility that negative symptoms might also be part of the clinical presentation of the subgroup of psychotic bipolar cases that are particularly likely to carry the dysbindin risk haplotype.

G72 (DAOA)/G30

This locus was first implicated in studies of schizophrenia by Chumakov and colleagues,[42] who undertook association mapping in the linkage region on chromosome 13q22–34. They found associations in French Canadian and Russian populations in markers around two novel, putative genes, *G72* and *G30*, which are overlapping but transcribed in opposite directions. Both *G72* and *G30* are apparently transcribed in brain, but in vitro translation experiments only resulted in production of protein for *G72*. Yeast two-hybrid analysis of experimentally produced protein provided evidence for physical interaction between G72 and D-amino acid oxidase *(DAO)*. DAO is expressed in human brain where it oxidizes D-serine, a potent activator of *N*-methyl-D-aspartate glutamate receptor. Coincubation of G72 and DAO in vitro revealed a functional interaction with G72 enhancing the activity of DAO. Consequently, G72 has now been named D-amino acid oxidase activator (DAOA). However, it should be noted that the existence of native G72 protein has not been demonstrated and there have been, as yet, no reports replicating the physical interaction with DAO. Associations between schizophrenia and markers in and around *DAOA* have subsequently been reported by a number of groups and supported by recent meta-analysis,[43] although once again there is no consensus concerning the specific risk alleles or haplotypes across studies. Moreover, unlike *NRG1* and *DTNBP1*, this locus has been quite extensively studied in bipolar disorder, for which it is now arguably the best-supported locus. Support for association with bipolar disorder has been reported from at least five independent data sets, and, as for schizophrenia, the presence of association is supported by meta-analysis without clear implication of specific alleles or haplotypes.[43] No pathologically relevant variant has yet been identified, and the biological mechanism remains to be elucidated.

The largest study to date, and the only one which has attempted to tag all common genetic variation at this locus, was published after the meta-analysis of Detera-Wadleigh and McMahon[43] was completed. This included 2,831 individuals, of whom 709 had DSM-IV schizophrenia, 706 had bipolar I disorder, and 1,416 were ethnically matched controls.[44] The authors identified significant association with bipolar disorder but failed to find association with schizophrenia. Analyses across the traditional diagnostic categories revealed significant evidence for association in the subset of cases ($n = 818$) in which episodes of major mood disorder had occurred. A similar pattern of association was observed in both bipolar cases and schizophrenia cases in which individuals had experienced major mood disorder. In contrast, there was no evidence for association in the subset of cases ($n = 1,153$) in which psychotic features occurred. This finding requires replication, but the data as they stand suggest that, despite being originally reported as a schizophrenia susceptibility locus, variation in *DAOA/G30* does not primarily increase susceptibility for prototypical schizophrenia or psychosis. Instead, it appears that variation in *DAOA/G30* influences susceptibility to episodes of mood disorder across the traditional bipolar and schizophrenia categories. Importantly, these findings also imply that whether or not significant associations are seen in schizophrenia will depend upon the proportion of cases that have suffered from episodes of mood disorder and remind us of the potential importance of sample differences in determining the reproducibility of genetic association studies.

Disrupted in Schizophrenia 1

This gene was implicated through studies of an extended pedigree in which a balanced chromosomal translocation (1;11)(q42;q14.3) showed strong evidence for linkage to a fairly broad phenotype comprising schizophrenia, bipolar disorder, and recurrent depression.[45] The translocation was found to disrupt two genes on chromosome 1: *DISC1* and *DISC2*.[45,46] *DISC2* contains no open reading frame and may regulate *DISC1* expression via antisense RNA.[46] A small pedigree has recently been reported in which a 4-bp deletion in exon 12 of *DISC1* cosegregates with schizophrenia and schizoaffective disorder,[47] although independent evidence suggests that the deletion is unlikely to be a highly penetrant risk allele for psychosis.[48] Interestingly, *DISC1* and *DISC2* are located close to the chromosome 1 markers implicated in two Finnish linkage studies of schizophrenia.[49,50] The Edinburgh group that identified *DISC1* found no linkage evidence in their own schizophrenia sample but did find suggestive evidence for linkage in bipolar disorder.[51] More recently, Hamshere and colleagues[30] reported genome-wide significant evidence for linkage at this locus in a linkage study of schizoaffective disorder, bipolar type. *DISC1* is certainly an interesting candidate gene for mental disorder, but it is important to remember that translocations exert effects on genes other than those directly disrupted. For example, there are several mechanisms by which a translocation can influence the expression of neighboring genes. In order to unequivocally implicate *DISC1* and/or *DISC2* in the pathogenesis of psychosis, it is necessary to identify mutations or polymorphisms that are associated with psychosis in nondeleted cases and are not in linkage disequilibrium with neighboring genes. Negative studies in schizophrenia samples were initially reported by the Edinburgh group with a small number of markers[52] and by a group who focused on the 5' end of the gene in a large Japanese sample.[53] More recently, several groups have reported positive findings,[54–57] although in no case are the results compelling and there is little agreement as to the specific markers or haplotypes showing association. Interestingly, in three of these studies, associations were observed with bipolar disorder as well as schizophrenia,[54–56] and in one the strongest association was observed with schizoaffective disorder.[55]

While no consistent pattern of association has yet emerged and no pathogenically relevant variants have been established, the convergence of the linkage data is strongly suggestive that variation in *DISC1* or another gene in this region influences susceptibility to mood-psychosis phenotypes that cut across the traditional Kraepelinian divide.

Conclusions

Genetic epidemiological data are beginning to favor the view that schizophrenia, bipolar disorder, and schizoaffective disorders share at least some genetic liability, although more work aimed at exploring these issues in adequately powered and suitably designed family and twin studies is clearly needed. Recent work on specific candidate genes supports this view and suggests that the genetic associations are strongest with clinical syndromes that do not map directly onto either or both of the two hypothetical disease entities proposed by Kraepelin. This is not surprising, given the frequency with which clinicians encounter mixed forms and the absence of a clear demarcation or "zone of rarity" between the two syndromes.[58] It also seems congruent with the evidence that schizophrenia and bipolar disorder share a range of other risk factors.[7] Moreover, general medicine provides multiple examples of genetically complex disorders where distinct diagnostic categories (e.g., hypertension, hemorrhagic stroke, myocardial infarction, and hypertensive cardiomyopathy) share genetic risk factors.[59]

The comparative work on candidate genes in the major psychiatric disorders is still in its early stages, and the findings should be treated with caution until further studies have been reported, given the difficulties in establishing unequivocal evidence for genetic association in complex diseases and the fact that for none of the genes implicated have specific risk variants so far been established. Indeed, it may turn out that many of the candidate genes currently discussed contain multiple risk (and protective) variants with effects on different aspects of psychopathology. A more parsimonious interpretation of the existing data is that variation in *DISC1/DISC2* and *NRG1* can confer predisposition to illness in individuals on either side of the Kraepelinian divide and that the effects of both genes will be felt most strongly in disorders with features of both schizophrenia and bipolar disorder. Variation in *DTNBP1* seems to predominantly predispose to schizophrenia and negative symptoms, with an effect on bipolar disorder confined to those cases with prominent psy-

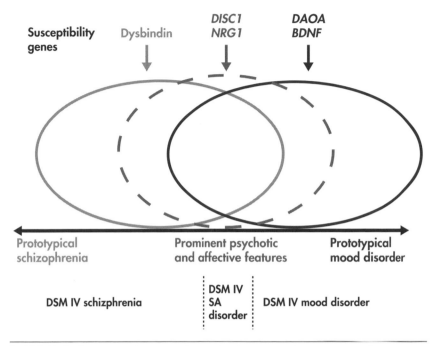

FIGURE 6–1. Simplified hypothesized relationship between specific suscepti-bility genes *(above the black line)* and clinical phenotype *(below the line)* using the model outlined in Craddock and Owen.[5]

The overlapping ellipses represent overlapping sets of genes: *light gray* influencing susceptibility to phenotypes with prominent schizophrenia-like features, *black* to prominent mood features, and *dashed* to phenotypes with a prominent mix of both types of feature. These assignments are based on current data and are likely to require revision as more data accumulate.

chotic features. In contrast, *DAOA/G30* appears to be more strongly associated with mood disorder, and the extent to which associations with schizophrenia are seen may depend upon the proportion of cases with prominent mood disorder features.

Such findings will have important implications for future classifications of the major psychiatric disorders because they suggest an overlap in the biological basis of disorders that have, over the past 100 years, been regarded as distinct entities.[5] We predict that, over the coming years, molecular genetics will catalyze a reap-praisal of psychiatric nosology as well as contribute in a major way to our under-standing of the pathophysiology and the development of improved treatments. Current genetic findings suggest that rather than classifying psychosis as a dichot-omy, a more useful formulation may be to conceptualize alternative categories or a spectrum of clinical phenotypes with susceptibility conferred by overlapping sets of genes[5] (Figure 6–1).

For the time being, however, such interpretations remain largely speculative as our understanding of the brain mechanisms linking specific gene actions and products to the subjective experience of psychopathological symptoms, such as delusions, hallucinations, or thought disorder, is at best rudimentary. There is an "explanatory gap" between the findings of statistical association of a gene variant with the disorder and the demonstration of *causality* with regard to specific illness phenomena. This gap might be easier to bridge by employing intermediate (or endo-) phenotypes in the domains of cognition, neurophysiology, or neuroanatomy. As objectively measurable quantitative traits, endophenotypes are better anchored in brain biology than clinical symptoms and can help delineate subtypes of disorder with likely distinct genetic basis.[60,61] The dissection of the syndromes of psychosis into "modular" endophenotypes with specific neurocognitive or neurophysiological underpinnings, cutting across the conventional diagnostic boundaries, is beginning to be perceived as a promising approach in the genetics of the major psychiatric disorders.[62]

It is important that researchers are willing to embrace and explore such alternative approaches to the phenotype of psychosis in order to interpret the accumulating data and design new research. This will be an iterative process with identified genetic signals allowing refinement of the phenotype and the refined phenotype allowing increased power to detect further genetic signals. To facilitate this approach, it will be important to collect large samples that have a full representation of phenotypes across the mood-psychosis spectrum and detailed, high-quality phenotypic assessments, preferably including dimensional measures (e.g., Levinson et al.,[63] Craddock et al.[64]).

In conclusion, accumulating evidence supports the existence of an overlap in genetic susceptibility across the traditional Kraepelinian divide with studies of several genes providing to date the most compelling such evidence. This work is at an early stage but has the potential to change our conception of psychiatric nosology as well as our understanding of the pathogenesis of psychopathology.

References

1. American Psychiatric Association. Diagnostic and Statistical Manual of Mental Disorders. 4th ed. Washington, DC: American Psychiatric Association; 1994.
2. World Health Organization. The ICD-10 Classification of Mental and Behavioural Disorders. Diagnostic Criteria for Research. Geneva, Switzerland: World Health Organization; 1993.
3. Kraepelin E. Patterns of mental disorders. In: Hirsch SR, Shepherd M, eds. Themes and Variations in European Psychiatry. Bristol, England: John Wright and Sons; 1974:7–30.
4. American Psychiatric Association. Diagnostic and Statistical Manual of Mental Disorders. 3rd ed. Washington, DC: American Psychiatric Association; 1980.

5. Craddock N, Owen MJ. The beginning of the end for the Kraepelinian dichotomy. Br J Psychiatry. 2005;186:364–366.
6. van Os J, Gilvarry C, Bale R, et al. A comparison of the utility of dimensional and categorical representations of psychosis. UK700 group. Psychol Med. 1999;29:595–606.
7. Murray RM, Sham P, Van Os J, Zanelli J, Cannon M, McDonald C. A developmental model for similarities and dissimilarities between schizophrenia and bipolar disorder. Schizophr Res. 2004;71:405–416.
8. Gottesman II. Schizophrenia Genesis: The Origins of Madness. New York: Freeman; 1991.
9. Tsuang MT, Faraone SV. The Genetics of Mood Disorders. Baltimore, MD: The Johns Hopkins University Press; 1990.
10. Baron M, Gruen R, Asnis L, et al. Schizoaffective illness, schizophrenia and affective disorders: morbidity risk and genetic transmission. Acta Psychiatr Scand. 1982;65:253–262.
11. Gershon ES, Hamovit J, Guroff JJ, et al. A family study of schizoaffective, bipolar I, bipolar II, unipolar, and normal control probands. Arch Gen Psychiatry. 1982;39:1157–1167.
12. Frangos E, Athanassenas G, Tsitourides S, et al. Prevalence of DSM III schizophrenia among the first-degree relatives of schizophrenic probands. Acta Psychiatr Scand. 1985;72:382–386.
13. Gershon ES, DeLisi LE. A controlled family study of chronic psychoses: schizophrenia and schizoaffective disorder. Arch Gen Psychiatry. 1988;45:328–336.
14. Kendler KS, McGuire M, Gruenberg AM, et al. The Roscommon family study: affective-illness, anxiety disorder, and alcoholism in relatives. Arch Gen Psychiatry. 1993;50:952–960.
15. Maier W, Lichtermann D, Minges J, et al. Continuity and discontinuity of affective-disorders and schizophrenia: results of a controlled family study. Arch Gen Psychiatry. 1993;50:871–883.
16. Tsuang MT, Winokur G, Crowe RR. Morbidity risks of schizophrenia and affective disorders among first degree relatives of patients with schizophrenia, mania, depression and surgical conditions. Br J Psychiatry. 1980;137:497–504.
17. Valles V, Van Os J, Guillamat R, et al. Increased morbid risk for schizophrenia in families of in-patients with bipolar illness. Schizophr Res. 2000;42:83–90.
18. Pope HG Jr, Yurgelun-Todd D. Schizophrenic individuals with bipolar first-degree relatives: analysis of two pedigrees. J Clin Psychiatry. 1990;51:97–101.
19. Kendler KS, Karkowski LM, Walsh D. The structure of psychosis: latent class analysis of probands from the Roscommon family study. Arch Gen Psychiatry. 1998;55:492–499.
20. Rice J, Reich T, Andreasen NC, et al. The familial transmission of bipolar illness. Arch Gen Psychiatry. 1987;44:441–447.
21. Osby U, Brandt L, Terenius L. The risk for schizophrenia and bipolar disorder in siblings to probands with schizophrenia and bipolar disorder. Am J Med Genet. 2001;105:O56.
22. Slater E, Shields J. Psychotic and Neurotic Illnesses in Twins. Medical Research Council Special Report 278. London: Her Majesty's Stationery Office; 1953.

23. Slater E, Cowle V. The Genetics of Mental Disorders. London: Oxford University Press; 1971.
24. Farmer AE, McGuffin P, Gottesman II. Twin concordance for DSM-III schizophrenia: scrutinizing the validity of the definition. Arch Gen Psychiatry. 1987;44:634–641.
25. Cardno AG, Rijsdijk FV, Sham PC, et al. A twin study of genetic relationships between psychotic symptoms. Am J Psychiatry. 2002;159:539–545.
26. McGuffin P, Reveley A, Holland A. Identical triplets: nonidentical psychosis? Br J Psychiatry. 1982;140:1–6.
27. Badner JA, Gershon ES. Meta-analysis of whole-genome linkage scans of bipolar disorder and schizophrenia. Mol Psychiatry. 2002;7:405–411.
28. Berrettini W. Evidence for shared susceptibility in bipolar disorder and schizophrenia. Am J Med Genet. 2003;123C:59–64.
29. Craddock N, O'Donovan MC, Owen MJ. The genetics of schizophrenia and bipolar disorder: dissecting psychosis. J Med Genet. 2005;42:193–204.
30. Hamshere ML, Bennett P, Williams N, et al. Genome-wide linkage scan in schizoaffective disorder: significant evidence for linkage (LOD= 3.54) at 1q42 close to DISC1, and suggestive evidence at 22q11 and 19q13. Arch Gen Psychiatry. 2005;62:1081–1088.
31. Craddock N, Owen MJ, O'Donovan MC. The catechol-O-methyltransferase gene (COMT) as a candidate for psychiatric phenotypes: evidence and lessons. Mol Psychiatry. 2006;11:446–458.
32. Stefansson H, Sigurdsson E, Steinthorsdottir V, et al. Neuregulin 1 and susceptibility to schizophrenia. Am J Hum Genet. 2002;71:877–892.
33. Stefansson H, Sarginson J, Kong A, et al. Association of neuregulin 1 with schizophrenia confirmed in a Scottish population. Am J Hum Genet. 2003;72:83–87.
34. Williams NM, Norton N, Williams H, et al. A systematic genome-wide linkage study in 353 sib pairs with schizophrenia. Am J Hum Genet. 2003;73:1355–1367.
35. Tosato S, Dazzan P, Collier D. Association between the neuregulin 1 gene and schizophrenia: a systematic review. Schizophr Bull. 2005;31:613–617.
36. Green E, Raybould R, McGregor S, et al. The operation of the schizophrenia susceptibility gene, neuregulin 1 (NRG1) across traditional diagnostic boundaries to increase risk for bipolar disorder. Arch Gen Psychiatry. 2005;62:642–648.
37. Straub RE, Jiang Y, MacLean CJ, et al. Genetic variation in the 6p22.3 gene DTNBP1, the human ortholog of the mouse dysbindin gene, is associated with schizophrenia. Am J Hum Genet. 2002;71:337–348.
38. Williams NM, O'Donovan MC, Owen MJ. Is the dysbindin gene (DTNBP1) a susceptibility gene for schizophrenia? Schizophr Bull. 2005;31:800–805.
39. Raybould R, Green EK, MacGregor S, et al. Bipolar disorder and polymorphisms in the dysbindin (dystrobrevin binding protein 1) gene (DTNBP1). Biol Psychiatry. 2005;57:696–701.
40. Breen G, Prata D, Osborne S, et al. Association of the dysbindin gene with bipolar affective disorder. Am J Psychiatry. 2006;163:1636–1638.
41. Fanous AH, van den Oord EJ, Riley BP, et al. Relationship between a high-risk haplotype in the DTNBP1 (dysbindin) gene and clinical features of schizophrenia. Am J Psychiatry. 2005;162:1824–1832.

42. Chumakov I, Blumenfeld M, Guerassimenko O, et al. Genetic and physiological data implicating the new human gene G72 and the gene for D-amino acid oxidase in schizophrenia. Proc Natl Acad Sci USA. 2002;99:13675–13680.
43. Detera-Wadleigh SD, McMahon FJ. G72/G30 in schizophrenia and bipolar disorder: review and meta-analysis. Biol Psychiatry. 2006;60:106–114.
44. Williams NM, Green EK, Macgregor S, et al. Variation at the DAOA/G30 locus influences susceptibility to major mood episodes but not psychosis in schizophrenia and bipolar disorder. Arch Gen Psychiatry. 2006;63:366–373.
45. Blackwood DH, Fordyce A, Walker MT, et al. Schizophrenia and affective disorders—cosegregation with a translocation at chromosome 1q42 that directly disrupts brain-expressed genes: clinical and P300 findings in a family. Am J Hum Genet. 2001;69:428–433.
46. Millar JK, Wilson-Annan JC, Anderson S, et al. Disruption of two novel genes by a translocation co-segregating with schizophrenia. Hum Mol Genet. 2000;9:1415–1423.
47. Sachs NA, Sawa A, Holmes SE, Ross CA, DeLisi LE, Margolis RL. A frameshift mutation in Disrupted in Schizophrenia 1 in an American family with schizophrenia and schizoaffective disorder. Mol Psychiatry. 2005;10:758–764.
48. Green E, Norton N, Peirce T, et al. Evidence that a DISC1 frame-shift deletion associated with psychosis in a single family may not be a pathogenic mutation. Mol Psychiatry. 2006;11:798–799.
49. Ekelund J, Hovatta I, Parker A, et al. Chromosome 1 loci in Finnish schizophrenia families. Hum Mol Genet. 2001;10:1611–1617.
50. Ekelund J, Hennah W, Hiekkalinna T, et al. Replication of 1q42 linkage in Finnish schizophrenia pedigrees. Mol Psychiatry. 2004;9:1037–1041.
51. Macgregor S, Visscher PM, Knott SA, et al. A genome scan and follow-up study identify a bipolar disorder susceptibility locus on chromosome 1q42. Mol Psychiatry. 2004;9:1083–1090.
52. Devon RS, Anderson S, Teague PW, et al. Identification of polymorphisms within Disrupted in Schizophrenia 1 and Disrupted in Schizophrenia 2, and an investigation of their association with schizophrenia and bipolar disorder. Psychiatr Genet. 2002;11:71–78.
53. Kockelkorn TT, Arai M, Matsumoto H, et al. Association study of polymorphisms in the 5' upstream region of human DISC1 gene with schizophrenia. Neurosci Lett. 2004;368:41–45.
54. Hennah W, Varilo T, Kestila M, et al. Haplotype transmission analysis provides evidence of association for DISC1 to schizophrenia and suggests sex-dependent effects. Hum Mol Genet. 2003;12:3151–3159.
55. Hodgkinson CA, Goldman D, Jaeger J, et al. Disrupted in schizophrenia 1 (DISC1): association with schizophrenia, schizoaffective disorder, and bipolar disorder. Am J Hum Genet. 2004;75:862–872.
56. Thomson PA, Wray NR, Millar JK, et al. Association between the TRAX/DISC locus and both bipolar disorder and schizophrenia in the Scottish population. Mol Psychiatry. 2005;10:657–668, 616.

57. Callicott JH, Straub RE, Pezawas L, et al. Variation in DISC1 affects hippocampal structure and function and increases risk for schizophrenia. Proc Natl Acad Sci USA. 2005;102:8627–8632.

58. Kendell R, Jablensky A. Distinguishing between the validity and utility of psychiatric diagnoses. Am J Psychiatry. 2003;160:4–12.

59. Kendler KS. Reflections on the relationship between psychiatric genetics and psychiatric nosology. Am J Psychiatry. 2006;163:1138–1146.

60. Hallmayer JF, Kalaydjieva L, Badcock J, et al. Genetic evidence for a distinct subtype of schizophrenia characterized by pervasive cognitive deficit. Am J Hum Genet. 2005;77:468–476.

61. Jablensky A. Subtyping schizophrenia: implications for genetic research. Mol Psychiatry. 2006;11:815–836.

62. Harrison PJ, Owen MJ. Genes for schizophrenia? Recent findings and their pathophysiological implications. Lancet. 2003;361:417–419.

63. Levinson DF, Mowry BJ, Escamilla MA, Faraone SV. The Lifetime Dimensions of Psychosis Scale (LDPS): description and interrater reliability. Schizophr Bull. 2002;28:683–695.

64. Craddock N, Jones I, Kirov G, et al. The Bipolar Affective Disorder Dimension Scale (BADDS)—a dimensional scale for rating lifetime psychopathology in bipolar spectrum disorders. BMC Psychiatry. 2004;4:19.

7

HOW SHOULD DSM-V CRITERIA FOR SCHIZOPHRENIA INCLUDE COGNITIVE IMPAIRMENT?

Richard S. E. Keefe, Ph.D.
Wayne S. Fenton, M.D.

Neurocognitive deficits of schizophrenia are profound and clinically relevant. Patients with schizophrenia perform 1.5–2.0 standard deviations (SDs) below healthy control subjects on a variety of neurocognitive tasks. The most prominent of these deficits are memory, attention, working memory, problem solving, processing speed, and social cognition.[1] These impairments exist prior to the initiation of antipsychotic treatment[2] and are not caused by psychotic symptoms in patients who are able to complete cognitive testing, which includes the overwhelming majority

Reprinted with permission from Keefe RSE, Fenton WS. "How Should DSM-V Criteria for Schizophrenia Include Cognitive Impairment?" *Schizophrenia Bulletin* 2007; 33: 912–920.

This article was generated from a meeting on "Deconstructing Psychosis" at the offices of the American Psychiatric Association in Arlington, VA, on February 16–17, 2006. In that meeting, Dr. Keefe presented many of the ideas discussed in this article, and they were commented on formally by Dr. Fenton and informally by other panel participants. While Dr. Fenton agreed to coauthor this article, he was not able to make comments on the manuscript before his tragic death on September 2, 2006.

of patients.[3] The various cognitive deficits in schizophrenia have all been shown to be associated with functional outcomes such as difficulty with community functioning, difficulty with instrumental and problem-solving skills, reduced success in psychosocial rehabilitation programs,[4] and the inability to maintain successful employment.[5] In fact, cognitive deficits are better able to explain important functional outcomes, such as work performance and independent living,[6] than positive or negative symptoms.

The importance of cognitive deficits in schizophrenia goes beyond their severity and relation to functional outcomes. Cognitive deficits appear to be present in some patients with schizophrenia prior to the onset of psychosis and are correlated with measurable brain dysfunction more than any other aspect of the illness. While the number of studies associating negative or positive symptoms with abnormal brain imaging results is small, the imaging literature in schizophrenia is filled with associations between cognitive deficits and structural and functional imaging results that differ from healthy control subjects. Perhaps most importantly, cognition is increasingly considered as a primary target for treatment.[7-10]

Despite the relevance of cognitive impairment to biology, function, and treatment in schizophrenia, it is not included in the *Diagnostic and Statistical Manual of Mental Disorders,* 4th Edition (DSM-IV),[11] criteria. It is noteworthy, however, that the first [paragraph] of the description of schizophrenia in DSM-IV includes four references to cognitive disturbances [emphasis added]: "the characteristics of schizophrenia involve a range of *cognitive* and emotional dysfunctions that include perception, inferential thinking, language and communication, *behavioral monitoring,* affect, *fluency,* and production of thought and speech, hedonic capacity, volition and drive, and *attention.*"[11] Thus, it is clear that cognition is deemed important by diagnostic experts; however, a method for including this fundamental aspect of the illness in the diagnostic criteria for schizophrenia has not been determined. The current review will emphasize the importance of cognition in schizophrenia and forward a proposal for consideration that severe cognitive impairment should be part of the criteria for schizophrenia in *Diagnostic and Statistical Manual of Mental Disorders,* 5th Edition (DSM-V). A research agenda for determining the validity and usefulness of including cognitive impairment as part of the criteria for schizophrenia will be discussed.

Will Cognitive Impairment Help Distinguish the Diagnosis of Schizophrenia From Affective Disorders?

The first question that will be considered is whether adding some definition of cognitive impairment or cognitive decline to the criteria for schizophrenia will help define

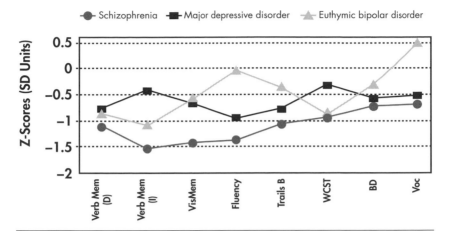

FIGURE 7–1. Cognitive profiles in schizophrenia, major depression, and euthymic bipolar disorder from published meta-analyses.[16]

Healthy group mean=0. BD=Wechsler Adult Intelligence Scale (WAIS) block design test; Trails B=Trail Making Test, B; Verb Mem (D)=delayed verbal memory; VerbMem (I)=immediate verbal memory; Vis Mem=visual memory; Voc=WAIS vocabulary; WCST=Wisconsin Card Sorting Test.

Source. Data from Heinrichs and Zakzanis,[44] Zakzanis et al.,[14] and van Gorp et al.[15] Reprinted from Buchanan et al.[10] with permission from Oxford University Press.

a "point of rarity" with affective psychoses.[12] The ability of a diagnostic refinement to improve the distinction between two entities and thus create an increased nonoverlap between them is considered to be a crucial determinant for inclusion.

DIAGNOSTIC DIFFERENCES IN SEVERITY OF COGNITIVE IMPAIRMENT

The conclusions from cognitive experts in the Measurement and Treatment Research to Improve Cognition in Schizophrenia (MATRICS) project were that "schizophrenia and schizoaffective disorder share a similar pattern of cognitive impairments, which is distinct from patterns in major depression, bipolar disorder, and Alzheimer's dementia."[10] This group of experts came to this conclusion based upon a series of studies indicating that patients with schizophrenia have a pattern of deficits that is more profound than those in major depression and bipolar disorder, more stable over the course of illness, and more related to clinical state. Meta-analyses of the cognitive profiles of patients with schizophrenia, major depression, and bipolar disorder are described in Figure 7–1. Patients with schizophrenia have more cognitive impairment on all the cognitive tests that were measured in each of the diagnostic groups. While the pattern of deficits among these groups may not differ dramatically, it is well accepted that the deficits of schizophrenia are more profound than those in affective disorders.[10,13] A recent meta-analysis comparing the performances of patients with schizophrenia and bipolar disorder concluded that patients with schizophrenia have cognitive deficits that are about 0.5 SD larger than those in patients with bipolar disorder. These deficits were found to be particularly profound on tests of verbal fluency, working memory, executive control, visual memory, mental speed, and verbal memory.[13] Even when patients with schizophrenia and patients with bipolar disorder were matched on the severity of their clinical symptoms, the deficits of schizophrenia surpassed those of patients with bipolar disorder by 0.5 SD.[13]

Studies of patients with first-episode schizophrenia and affective disorder appear to support the meta-analyses completed on more chronic patients. In an epidemiological study of all first-admission psychotic disorders in Suffolk County, NY, patients who received a diagnosis of schizophrenia at 24 months of follow-up ($n = 148$) were found to have significantly greater cognitive deficits compared with those first-episode psychotic patients who were diagnosed with bipolar disorder ($n = 87$) and depression ($n = 56$) 24 months later. Again, the differentiation between schizophrenia and affective psychoses was particularly profound with regard to memory, executive functions, and mental speed tasks (A. Reichenberg, Ph.D., unpublished data, 2007). These data suggest that cognitive information at first episode may aid in the determination of whether an individual's later diagnosis will be in the affective or schizophrenia spectrum.

DIAGNOSTIC DIFFERENCES REGARDING RELATION OF COGNITIVE IMPAIRMENT TO CLINICAL STATE

While patients with affective psychoses also have cognitive impairment, it appears as though these cognitive deficits are more strongly associated with clinical symptoms and state-related factors than in patients with schizophrenia.[14,15] In a study of patients with schizophrenia or bipolar disorder who were assessed when psychotic at baseline and then 8 months later, patients who were psychotic at follow-up in both diagnostic groups had no difference in their cognitive impairment 8 months later. Among those patients whose psychosis had remitted 8 months later, schizophrenia patients also showed the same level of cognitive impairment. Only the bipolar patients whose psychosis had remitted at follow-up had improved in their cognitive performance.[16] Similar data have been reported in first-episode samples. While first-episode patients with affective psychoses performed similarly to those with first-episode schizophrenia in one study, patients with nonpsychotic affective disorders performed significantly better than both psychotic groups.[17] Thus, while the cognitive deficits of affective disorders may be profound in some cases, these cognitive deficits appear to be related to clinical symptoms. In contrast, cognitive impairment in schizophrenia patients has

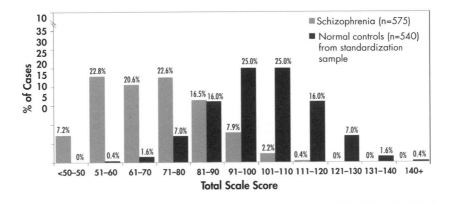

FIGURE 7–2. Distributions of total scores on the Repeatable Battery for the Assessment of Neuropsychological Status in patients with schizophrenia and healthy control subjects from published norms.

Source. Data from Randolph et al.[22] and Wilk et al.[23]

been repeatedly demonstrated to be uncorrelated with psychotic symptoms.[3,18–20] Part of the explanation for these low correlations between cognitive deficits and symptoms in patients with schizophrenia is that while the symptoms of schizophrenia wax and wane in almost all patients, leading to low stability coefficients over time,[21] the stability of cognitive deficits in all domains is very high, with test-retest coefficients ranging between 0.7 and 0.85 even in patients tested 1 year apart following their initial treatment for psychosis.[21] Thus, while there are cognitive deficits in affective disorders, they fluctuate in parallel with clinical symptom changes. In schizophrenia, however, they may be the most stable aspect of the disorder.

PREVALENCE OF COGNITIVE IMPAIRMENT IN SCHIZOPHRENIA

If cognitive impairment is to be considered as part of the diagnosis of schizophrenia, it will be important to demonstrate that its prevalence among patients with schizophrenia is high. Patients with schizophrenia and healthy control subjects both show normal distributions of scores on cognitive batteries such as the Repeatable Battery for the Assessment of Neuropsychological Status[22] (see Figure 7–2). However, as has been frequently demonstrated, the distribution of a large number of patients with schizophrenia (*n*=575) is shifted about 2 SDs below the 540 healthy control subjects from the standardization sample.[22,23] While there is considerable overlap between these two distributions, it is noteworthy that there are very few healthy control subjects at the lower ends of this distribution and very few schizophrenia patients at the upper ends of this distribution. Traditional neuropsychological criteria for cognitive impairment would identify those individuals

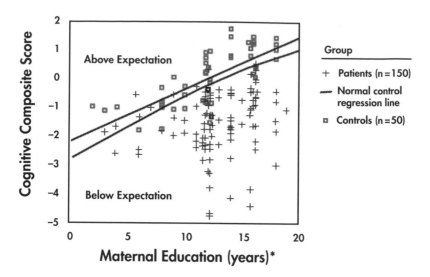

*Maternal education values jittered for clarity.

FIGURE 7–3.   Expected neurocognitive performance based on maternal education of healthy control subjects.

Source.   Reprinted from Keefe et al.[27] Copyright (2005), with permission from Elsevier.

who performed better than 1 SD below the healthy control mean as "unimpaired."[24–26] By these criteria, about 20% of the patients in this study would be considered to have normal cognitive functions. However, it is possible that many of the individuals at the upper end of this schizophrenia distribution have demonstrated cognitive decline compared with what their cognitive functions would have been if they had never developed the illness. While this conjecture can never be proved, it is useful to investigate the relationship between antecedent factors, such as parental education and reading scores, and their relationship to current cognitive functions in patients with schizophrenia.

In healthy control subjects, current cognitive ability is strongly predicted by antecedent factors such as maternal education and reading score.[27] As demonstrated in Figure 7–3, the healthy control subjects whose mothers had greater education clearly had higher cognitive functions. The regression line in this figure describes the relationship between these two factors. Because of the natural variability of cognitive performance among healthy control subjects, about half of this distribution performs above expectations while half performs below expectations. However, an overwhelming majority of the patients with schizophrenia in this sample performed below the expectations established by antecedent factors, in this case, maternal education. Thus, it is likely that almost all schizophrenic patients have some measure of cognitive deficit compared with what their level of cognitive function would have been if they had never developed the illness.

EARLY COGNITIVE DECLINE IN SCHIZOPHRENIA?

While most patients with schizophrenia appear to show some cognitive decline based upon what would have been predicted by antecedent factors, it is also important to note that on average patients with schizophrenia start out at a lower baseline prior to the onset of the illness. Children who will eventually develop schizophrenia show cognitive impairment compared with healthy control subjects and children who later develop affective disorders.[28,29] However, individuals who will eventually develop schizophrenia also appear to show decline on scholastic measures between early childhood and late adolescence.[29] The presence of cognitive deficits or cognitive decline during adolescence has been found to predict the conversion to schizophrenia in various samples.[29–34] Thus, as depicted in Figure 7–4, patients with schizophrenia appear to begin life with cognitive performance that is slightly worse than their peers. As childhood progresses, cognitive performance tends to worsen in those children who will eventually develop schizophrenia. By the time psychosis develops in late adolescence or early adulthood, patients perform substantially worse than their healthy peers. While patients with affective disorders also demonstrate cognitive impairment in adulthood, it appears as though these individuals do not show impairment until the adult onset of their disorders.[28]

The literature review above supports the notion that the severity and longitudinal course of cognitive impairment in schizophrenia differ substantially from that found in patients with affective psychosis. Yet the question of whether including a criterion of cognitive impairment or cognitive decline from healthy premorbid levels in the diagnosis of schizophrenia will help define a "point of rarity" with affective psychoses remains unanswered. Research studies and analyses of existing databases are needed that address this question in large numbers of psychotic individuals with schizophrenia and affective disorders assessed on measures of cognition and symptoms. These studies will help determine whether the inclusion of a criterion for cognitive impairment in the diagnosis of schizophrenia will increase the point of rarity between these diagnostic entities.

How Can Cognitive Impairment Be Assessed for Diagnostic Purposes?

While formal cognitive testing appears to be very sensitive to the cognitive impairment in schizophrenia, the resources required to complete neuropsychological evaluations are prohibitive in various treatment settings. In fact, the diagnoses of Alzheimer disease and attention-deficit/hyperactivity disorder (ADHD), while be-

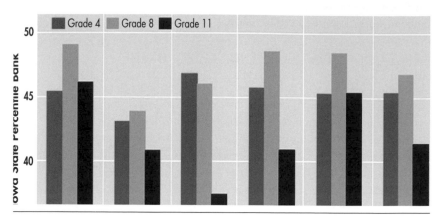

FIGURE 7–4.   Standardized scholastic test performance in grades 4, 8, and 11 relative to state norms for 70 subjects who later developed schizophrenia.

[a]Grade 4 and 8 results represent performance on the Iowa Tests of Basic Skills; grade 11 results represent performance on the Iowa Tests of Educational Development.

[b]Grade 11 score significantly lower than median percentile rank (F=5.89; df=1, 45; P<0.05).

[c]Grade 11 score significantly lower than median percentile rank (F=7.80; df=1, 45; P<0.01). Repeated measures ANOVA revealed a significant difference in scores among the three grades (F=3.18; df=2, 107; p<0.05), with further analyses showing that the grade 11 scores were significantly lower than the scores in grade 4 (F=5.04; df=1, 45; P<0.05) and grade 8 (F=4.97; df=1, 45; P<0.05).

[d]Grade 11 score significantly lower than median percentile rank (F=5.63; df=1, 45; P<0.05). Repeated measures ANOVA revealed a significant difference in scores among the three grades (F=3.66; df=2, 107; P<0.03), with further analyses showing that the grade 11 scores were significantly lower than the scores in grade 8 (F=6.40; df=1, 46; P=0.01).

[e]Grade 11 score significantly lower than median percentile rank (F=4.77; df=1, 45; P<0.05).

Source.   Reprinted with permission from Fuller et al.[29]

ing clearly cognitive disorders, do not require formal cognitive testing. Thus, it may not be realistic to expect that the diagnosis of schizophrenia would depend upon cognitive performance testing. It needs to be established how cognitive impairment will be assessed by clinicians who will diagnose schizophrenia so that the additional criterion will contribute sufficiently to diagnostic validity and treatment success. Recent work suggests that almost all the variance in cognitive composite scores can be accounted for by a small number of tests.[3] Thus, clinicians may be able to develop the capacity to assess cognitive impairment in schizophrenia without overwhelming resource requirements. However, education and training on the use of standardized cognitive tests for clinicians will be essential to assure that the assessment procedures are completed in a manner that maintains test standardization. This aspect of training is usually included in the curriculum of clinical psychologists and neuropsychologists but is rarely a component of education for physicians, social workers, and nurses. A program for training in cognitive testing will be an essential step to increase the capacity for clinicians to assess the cognitive impairments of schizophrenia. It will take time to work this training into the traditional education of psychiatrists and other nonpsychologists. This training does not need to be limited to formal neuropsychological tests but may be better aimed toward the assessment of patients' ability on practical cognitive tasks, which may have stronger direct correlations with outcome.[35]

INTERVIEW-BASED ASSESSMENTS OF COGNITION

While the lack of availability of formal test methods and trained testers may prohibit testing in many clinical environments, recent methodological advances have included the assessment of cognition in patients with schizophrenia with interview-based measures. Similar to ADHD assessment methods, which do not involve formal testing, these measures involve a series of questions directed toward the patient with schizophrenia and his or her relatives or caregivers. These questions address whether people with schizophrenia have cognitive deficits that impair fundamental aspects of their daily lives. For instance, some of the questions ask whether patients have difficulty remembering names, concentrating well enough to read a newspaper or book, being able to follow group conversations, and handling changes in daily routines.[36,37] Interview-based assessments of cognition have historically been unreliable and have demonstrated low correlations with cognitive performance. However, these measures have generally relied upon the reports from patients and their treating clinicians, which have been notoriously unreliable and potentially invalid.[38–41] A methodology that assesses cognition with interviews of patients and caregivers, such as relatives or caseworkers, may have improved reliability and validity. For example, the Schizophrenia Cognition Rating Scale (SCoRS) has been found to have excellent reliability and substantial correlations with cognitive performance and functional outcomes[36] (M.F. Green, Ph.D., unpublished data, 2007). In fact, SCoRS global outcome measures have met several of the criteria for coprimary measures outlined by the MATRICS meeting for optimal designs for cognitive enhancement trials.[10] One of the potential weaknesses of this methodology, however, is that reports from patients have been found to have reduced reliability if patients are the only source of information. The relevance of this weakness is particularly important in the assessment of patients with schizophrenia because a substantial percentage of patients do not have an available informant who can provide information about the patient's cognitive deficits and how these deficits affect the patient's daily behavior. For example, in the MATRICS Psychometric and Standardization Study (PASS), test-retest reliability data over the course of 1 month was high when ratings were based upon a patient and informant as a source of information (intraclass correlation

[ICC] = 0.82, goodness of fit [GF] = 123; P = 0.001) (M. F. Green, Ph.D., unpublished data, 2007). However, when patients were the only source of information, the test-retest reliability coefficient (ICC) was 0.60 (GF = 148, P < 0.001). While reliability is enhanced when information can be obtained from both sources, a considerable number of patients do not have an available informant. A more extensive series of questions, as found in the Clinical Global Impression of Cognition in Schizophrenia (CGI-CoGS),[37] appears to improve the reliability of patient reports up to ICC = 0.80, but patients describe these longer interviews, which require up to 45 minutes each, as burdensome (M. F. Green, Ph.D., unpublished data, 2007). A shorter, less burdensome instrument that would not require an informant and could be completed on almost all patients would be ideal, although is not currently available. Future studies should focus on this methodology and must also determine whether interview-based assessments of cognition can contribute to the diagnostic separation between schizophrenia and affective psychoses.

Is the Clinical Importance of Cognition in Schizophrenia Sufficient to Include It in the Formal Criteria?

Even if including a definition of "cognitive impairment" in the criteria for schizophrenia does not increase the point of rarity between schizophrenia and other psychotic disorders, an additional consideration is whether it would be able to "provide useful information not contained in the definition of the disorder that helps in decisions about management and treatment."[42] The inclusion of cognitive impairment in the criteria for schizophrenia may increase psychiatrists' attention toward a neglected aspect of the core components of schizophrenia.[7] Because cognition is rarely considered among psychiatrists as an important treatment target, inclusion of cognitive impairment in the criteria for schizophrenia may help to educate clinicians about the importance of cognition in their treatment options. Furthermore, representatives from the U.S. Food and Drug Administration (FDA) have indicated that the recognition of cognitive impairment in the diagnostic nomenclature would be an important step in approving a drug for a cognitive improvement indication.[10] Many government agencies and pharmaceutical companies are currently involved in intense work to try to develop compounds that may improve cognition with schizophrenia. If successful, these compounds have the potential to alter the way that schizophrenia is currently treated. However, if the pathway is not established to allow these medications to be approved by the FDA, and if clinicians are not trained to recognize cognitive improvement, this potential area of great benefit to patients may be missed. Inclusion of cognitive impairment in the diagnostic criteria for schizophrenia may be one of the steps that could be taken to help clinicians target and potentially improve cognition in patients with schizophrenia.

How Should Cognitive Impairment in Schizophrenia Be Defined?

We have presented an argument for the importance of cognitive impairment in schizophrenia and have suggested that cognitive impairment should be represented in the diagnosis for schizophrenia. However, there are several considerations regarding how it should be included. We propose that the following criterion should be considered for the diagnosis of schizophrenia: "a level of cognitive functioning suggesting a consistent severe impairment and/or a significant decline from premorbid levels considering the patient's educational, familial, and socioeconomic background." Diagnosticians should consider all aspects of cognitive impairment in this definition but should be alerted that, in general, schizophrenia patients may have particularly severe deficits in the cognitive domains of memory, attention, working memory, reasoning and problem solving, processing speed, and social cognition.[1] It is not uncommon for some aspects of cognition to be unimpaired in the context of severe impairments in other areas, with an overall level of impairment in the severe range. A statement that the assessment of cognitive function must consider the patients' background was included to avoid overdiagnosing schizophrenia in individuals whose environments deprive them of their ability to develop cognitive abilities. In the event that DSM-V changes to a completely dimensional approach to the symptoms of psychosis,[43] cognitive impairment should be one of the key dimensions.

This change in DSM will potentially increase the point of rarity with other psychoses. It is likely that some patients diagnosed with schizophrenia who have little or no cognitive impairment have treatment responses and courses of illness that are more consistent with a diagnosis of affective disorder. If this is the case, it will benefit clinicians to change their expectations based upon this revised diagnosis. On the other hand, some patients diagnosed with affective disorders and severe cognitive impairment may follow the longitudinal course and treatment response of patients with schizophrenia. One of the important research questions that will need to be addressed is whether patients whose diagnosis changes based upon the new criteria are more likely to have genetic and other biological indicators consistent with the new diagnosis.

Changing the DSM criteria for schizophrenia to include cognitive impairment will also force clinicians to consider the cognitive impairment of their patients, which has been largely ignored among clinical psychiatrists. This change would thus direct clinicians' attention toward the aspect of the disorder that is the largest determinant of long-term functioning. It may also help develop the pathway for new treatments to improve this fundamental component of the illness and force educational systems to teach clinicians how to recognize cognitive impairment and improvement.

However, the implementation of this change in DSM will present several challenges. If this criterion is included in the criteria for schizophrenia, it will be crucial to consider how cognition will be measured by clinicians and researchers making a diagnosis. It is unrealistic to expect that all patients with schizophrenia would receive formal neuropsychological testing by psychologists, which is time consuming and expensive. In most treatment settings, these costs are prohibitive. However, if cognitive paradigms were developed that were able definitively to separate diagnostic entities, a case could be made that this testing is essential to patient diagnosis and treatment planning. Unfortunately, as discussed above, we are not yet at this stage.

A second consideration regarding the use of cognitive impairment as a criterion for schizophrenia is that current cognitive performance is affected by factors unrelated to cognitive decline in patients with schizophrenia such as level of education and environments that are variably conducive to normal learning.[23] Some patients may have very poor cognitive functioning due to factors unrelated to schizophrenia, whereas other patients may have cognitive performance that is in the "normal range" despite significant decline from premorbid levels. How will diagnosticians determine how schizophrenia may interact with these factors to result in a patient's current cognitive levels? Since not all patients are defined as "impaired" on cognitive tests, it is important to emphasize that the criterion will be met if a patient's current cognitive performance represents a "decline from premorbid cognitive functioning." On average, the longitudinal course of cognitive function in patients with schizophrenia appears to decline at least one full standard deviation from childhood. During childhood and adolescence, patients who will eventually develop schizophrenia perform about 0.5 SD below their peers who will not develop schizophrenia.[28,29,31] Immediately prior to the onset of psychosis, patients who are about to develop schizophrenia demonstrate a worsened cognitive function, such that the average person at ultra high risk for schizophrenia disorders who will eventually convert to psychosis performs about 1 SD below healthy control subjects.[30,34] It will be important in these cases for diagnosticians to determine whether there has been a decline in cognitive functions from expected cognitive levels based upon antecedent factors such as parental education, early school performance, and reading level. It will be essential for diagnosticians to collect a complete history on the cognitive performance of each patient, including how the patient's current cognitive performance compares with early school performance and any academic, intelligence, or cognitive testing that was performed during premorbid and prodromal periods. Furthermore, a patient's level of cognitive performance will need to be compared with other members of the patient's family and sociocultural background, if available. In some cases, testing would benefit this assessment. In other cases, the amount of cognitive impairment in a patient would be clearly obvious and in direct contrast to early cognitive competence in an individual. Finally, because cognitive impairment in affective disorders in the context of clinical exacerbation may be difficult to distinguish from schizophrenia cross-sectionally, longitudinal assessment will be important for an accurate diagnosis. While this historical and longitudinal data collection may initially appear to add burden, if indeed the level and course of cognitive deficit is crucial not only to diagnosis but also to prognosis and treatment planning, it is likely that this "front-loading" of clinical care may actually reduce clinical burden in the form of improved treatment response and long-term functioning.

Third, while clinician judgment will be an important component of assessing cognition in schizophrenia, recent data suggest that clinicians cannot be the sole source of information for making this determination. The challenge that arises here is that many patients with schizophrenia will not have enough contact with other people for someone to be able to report reliably on their usual level of cognitive functioning. Patients without available informants will need to have additional assessments such as more extensive interviews or an actual cognitive assessment, which is the most informative method for collecting cognitive information about a patient.

As discussed above, if a patient is assessed during a period of clinical exacerbation, cognitive impairment may be very similar in patients with schizophrenia and those with affective psychoses.[10,14,15] Thus, for the patient to meet the criterion of cognitive impairment, it will be important for the cognitive deficits to be stable throughout a long period of illness. This would help to differentiate the cognitive impairment found in schizophrenia from those in affective psychoses. However, it will also result in delays in definitive diagnoses in cases where cognitive impairment is present in the context of symptom exacerbation.

In sum, we have recommended for consideration that a criterion for consistent severe cognitive impairment be added to the DSM diagnosis of schizophrenia. There are several challenges for this suggestion to meet acceptance by the research and clinical communities. Research is needed to determine if such a criterion will increase the point of rarity between schizophrenia and other diagnostic entities; if clinicians are able to assess cognition reliably with brief formal assessment instruments or interview-based methods; and if the inclusion of such a criterion will improve the value of the diagnosis of schizophrenia for prognosis and treatment outcomes.

References

1. Nuechterlein KH, Barch DM, Gold JM, Goldberg TE, Green MF, Heaton RK. Identification of separable cognitive factors in schizophrenia. Schizophr Res. 2004;72:29–39.
2. Saykin AJ, Shtasel DL, Gur RE, et al. Neuropsychological deficits in neuroleptic naive patients with first-episode schizophrenia. Arch Gen Psychiatry. 1994;51:124–131.

3. Keefe RSE, Bilder RM, Harvey PD, et al. Baseline neurocognitive deficits in the CATIE schizophrenia trial. Neuropsychopharmacology. 2006;31:2033–2046.

4. Green MF, Kern RS, Braff DL, Mintz J. Neurocognitive deficits and functional outcome in schizophrenia: are we measuring the "right stuff"? Schizophr Bull. 2000;26:119–136.

5. Bryson G, Bell MD. Initial and final work performance in schizophrenia: cognitive and symptom predictors. J Nerv Ment Dis. 2003;191:87–92.

6. Harvey PD, Howanitz E, Parrella M, et al. Symptoms, cognitive functioning, and adaptive skills in geriatric patients with lifelong schizophrenia: a comparison across treatment sites. Am J Psychiatry. 1998;155:1080–1086.

7. Hyman SE, Fenton WS. Medicine. What are the right targets for psychopharmacology? Science. 2003;299:350–351.

8. Gold JM. Cognitive deficits as treatment targets in schizophrenia. Schizophr Res. 2004;72:21–28.

9. Davidson M, Keefe RSE. Cognitive impairment as a target for pharmacological treatment in schizophrenia. Schizophr Res. 1995;17:123–129.

10. Buchanan RW, Davis M, Goff D, et al. A summary of the FDA-NIMH-MATRICS workshop on clinical trial designs for neurocognitive drugs for schizophrenia. Schizophr Bull. 2005;31:5–21.

11. American Psychiatric Association. Diagnostic and Statistical Manual of Mental Disorders. 4th ed. Washington, DC: American Psychiatric Association; 1994.

12. Kendell R, Jablensky A. Distinguishing between the validity and utility of psychiatric diagnoses. Am J Psychiatry. 2003;160:4–12.

13. Krabbendam L, Arts B, van Os J, Aleman A. Cognitive functioning in patients with schizophrenia and bipolar disorder: a quantitative review. Schizophr Res. 2005;80:137–149.

14. Zakzanis KK, Leach L, Kaplan E. On the nature and pattern of neurocognitive function in major depressive disorders. Neuropsychiatry Neuropsychol Behav Neurol. 1998;11:111–119.

15. van Gorp WG, Altshuler L, Theberge DC, Wilkins J, Dixon W. Cognitive impairment in euthymic bipolar patients with and without prior alcohol dependence. Arch Gen Psychiatry. 1998;55:41–46.

16. Harvey PD, Docherty NM, Serper MR, Rasmussen M. Cognitive deficits and thought disorder: II. An 8-month follow-up study. Schizophr Bull. 1990;16:147–156.

17. Albus M, Hubmann W, Wahlheim C, Sobizack N, Franz U, Mohr F. Contrasts in neuropsychological test profile between patients with first-episode schizophrenia and first-episode affective disorders. Acta Psychiatr Scand. 1996;94:87–93.

18. Addington J, Addington D. Neurocognitive and social functioning in schizophrenia: a 2.5 year follow-up study. Schizophr Res. 2000;44:47–56.

19. Hughes C, Kumari V, Soni W, et al. Longitudinal study of symptoms and cognitive function in chronic schizophrenia. Schizophr Res. 2003;59:137–146.

20. Strauss ME. Relations of symptoms to cognitive deficits in schizophrenia. Schizophr Bull. 1993;19:215–231.

21. Bilder RM, Goldman RS, Robinson D, et al. Neuropsychology of first-episode schizophrenia: initial characterization and clinical correlates. Am J Psychiatry. 2000;157:549–559.

22. Randolph C. RBANS Manual: Repeatable Battery for the Assessment of Neuropsychological Status. Lutz, FL: PAR; 1998.

23. Wilk CM, Gold JM, Humber K, Dickerson F, Fenton WS, Buchanan RW. Brief cognitive assessment in schizophrenia: normative data for the Repeatable Battery for the Assessment of Neuropsychological Status. Schizophr Res. 2004;70:175–186.

24. Bryson GJ, Silverstein ML, Nathan A, Stephen L. Differential rate of neuropsychological dysfunction in psychiatric disorders: comparison between the Halstead-Reitan and Luria- Nebraska batteries. Percept Mot Skills. 1993;76:305–306.

25. Heinrichs RW, Awad AG. Neurocognitive subtypes of chronic schizophrenia. Schizophr Res. 1993;9:49–58.

26. Palmer BW, Heaton RK, Paulsen JS, et al. Is it possible to be schizophrenic yet neuropsychologically normal? Neuropsychology. 1997;11:437–446.

27. Keefe RS, Eesley CE, Poe MP. Defining a cognitive function decrement in schizophrenia. Biol Psychiatry. 2005;57:688–691.

28. Cannon M, Caspi A, Moffitt TE, et al. Evidence for early childhood, pan-developmental impairment specific to schizphreniform disorder: results from a longitudinal birth cohort. Arch Gen Psychiatry 2002;59:449–456.

29. Fuller R, Nopoulos P, Arndt S, O'Leary D, Ho BC, Andreasen NC. Longitudinal assessment of premorbid cognitive functioning in patients with schizophrenia through examination of standardized scholastic test performance. Am J Psychiatry. 2002;159:1183–1189.

30. Reichenberg A, Weiser M, Rapp MA, et al. Elaboration on premorbid intellectual performance in schizophrenia: premorbid intellectual decline and risk for schizophrenia. Arch Gen Psychiatry. 2005;62:1297–1304.

31. Davidson M, Reichenberg A, Rabinowitz J, Weiser M, Kaplan Z, Mark M. Behavioral and intellectual markers for schizophrenia in apparently healthy male adolescents. Am J Psychiatry. 1999;156:1328–1335.

32. Brewer WJ, Wood SJ, McGorry PD, et al. Impairment of olfactory identification ability in individuals at ultra-high risk for psychosis who later develop schizophrenia. Am J Psychiatry. 2003;160:1790–1794.

33. Brewer WJ, Francey SM, Wood SJ, et al. Memory impairments identified in people at ultra-high risk for psychosis who later develop first-episode psychosis. Am J Psychiatry. 2005;162:71–78.

34. Keefe RSE, Perkins DO, Gu H, Zipursky RB, Christensen BK, Lieberman JA. A longitudinal study of neurocognitive function in individuals at-risk for psychosis. Schizophr Res. 2006;88:26–35.

35. Bowie CR, Reichenberg A, Patterson TL, Heaton RK, Harvey PD. Determinants of real-world functional performance in schizophrenia subjects: correlations with cognition, function, functional capacity, and symptoms. Am J Psychiatry. 2006;163:418–425.

36. Keefe RSE, Poe M, Walker TM, Kang JW, Harvey PD. The Schizophrenia Cognition Rating Scale (SCoRS): interview-based assessment and its relationship to cognition, real-world functioning and functional capacity. Am J Psychiatry. 2006;163:426–432.

37. Ventura J, Bilder R, Cienfuegos A, Boxer O. Interview based measures of cognition in schizophrenia. Biol Psychiatry. 2006;59:1715.

38. Moritz S, Ferahli S, Naber D. Memory and attention performance in psychiatric patients: lack of correspondence between clinician-rated and patient-rated functioning with neuropsychological test results. J Int Neuropsychol Soc 2004;10:623–633.

39. van den Bosch RJ, Rombouts RP. Causal mechanisms of subjective cognitive dysfunction in schizophrenic and depressed patients. J Nerv Ment Dis. 1998;186:364–368.

40. Harvey PD, Serper MR, White L, et al. The convergence of neuropsychological testing and clinical ratings of cognitive impairment in patients with schizophrenia. Compr Psychiatry. 2001;42:306–313.

41. Stip E, Caron J, Renaud S, Pampoulova T, Lecomte Y. Exploring cognitive complaints in schizophrenia: the subjective scale to investigate cognition in schizophrenia. Compr Psychiatry. 2003;44:331–340.

42. Spitzer RL. Values and assumptions in the development of DSM-III and DSM-III-R: an insider's perspective and a belated response to Sadler, Hulgus, and Agich's "On values in recent American psychiatric classification." J Nerv Ment Dis. 2001;189:351–359.

43. Carpenter WT. Schizophrenia: diagnostic class or domains of pathology. Schizophr Bull. 2007;33:203.

44. Heinrichs RW, Zakzanis KK. Neurocognitive deficit in schizophrenia: a quantitative review of the evidence. Neuropsychology. 1998;12:426–445.

8

SEARCHING FOR UNIQUE ENDOPHENOTYPES FOR SCHIZOPHRENIA AND BIPOLAR DISORDER WITHIN NEURAL CIRCUITS AND THEIR MOLECULAR REGULATORY MECHANISMS

Francine M. Benes, M.D., Ph.D.

Endophenotypes are "measurable components unseen by the unaided eye that exist along the pathway between disease and distal genotype."[1] The field of psychiatry is now faced with the challenge of identifying endophenotypes for each disorder that shows there is compelling evidence that a heritable component contributes to susceptibility. In reality, an endophenotype is a rather ill-defined construct that probably involves neurophysiological, biochemical, endocrinological, neuroanatomical, cognitive, and even psychological factors.[1] Schizophrenia was

Reprinted with permission from Benes FM. "Searching for Unique Endophenotypes for Schizophrenia and Bipolar Disorder Within Neural Circuits and Their Molecular Regulatory Mechanisms." *Schizophrenia Bulletin* 2007; 33: 932–936.

the first psychiatric disorder for which compelling evidence for heritability was obtained from comparative studies of first-degree relatives as well as monozygotic and dizygotic twin pairs.[2] It has become apparent that heritability of a disorder, such as schizophrenia, involves many different factors. The concept of the "endophenotype" provides a means of operationalizing the identification of these factors.

In psychiatric disorders, this is particularly difficult because there are well-known similarities among the clinical phenotypes for very different disorders. For example, in psychotic disorders, the presence of hallucinations and delusions and a beneficial response to neuroleptic drugs often belies the fact that there are distinctly different genotypes associated with schizophrenia and bipolar disorder. Indeed, a single genotype can theoretically give rise to different clinical phenotypes, if there are different environmental influences associated with one phenotype versus another.[1] An important step toward identifying specific genotypes for schizophrenia and bipolar disorder is to identify meaningful endophenotypes for the various psychotic disorders.

A combination of clinical, epidemiological, neurobiological, and genetic studies can be used to select and evaluate different candidate endophenotypes.[3] For example, a defect in the P50 auditory evoked potential gating deficit, reportedly abnormal in schizophrenia, has been associated with a dysregulation in the expression of the alpha 7 nicotinic receptor in hippocampal γ-aminobutyric acid (GABA) cells.[4] At the level of neural circuits and their constituent cells, there are probably many such molecular interactions that can be examined. These may involve the influence of mutated DNA for specific genes on the relative abundance of their transcripts or their posttranslationally modified protein products. Gene expression profiling provides a particularly powerful tool for studying endophenotypes because it provides a broad cross-sectional profile of many different aspects of neuronal cell functioning including receptors, ion channels, transduction, signaling, metabolism, and transcriptional pathways. If the respective molecular profiles in two disorders such as schizophrenia and bipolar disorder are fundamentally different from one another, they may potentially be related to complex traits like those observed in psychotic patients. As molecular strategies of this type are used in the study of postmortem brain, they may eventually help to point the way toward a molecular basis for defining genotype and rational treatment strategies.[5] In the discussion that follows, this idea is considered in more detail by reviewing specific findings obtained in microscopic and microarray studies of the limbic lobe in schizophrenia and bipolar disorder.

Preferential Abnormalities in Discrete Aspects of Limbic Lobe

Over the past 20 years, postmortem studies have suggested that the limbic lobe consisting of the cingulate gyrus, hippocampal formation, entorhinal cortex, and amygdala may play a central role in the pathophysiology of schizophrenia.[6–11] Specific abnormalities in these regions have been reported using a variety of quantitative microscopic approaches (for a review, see Benes[12]). Noteworthy is the fact that significant changes have been preferentially found within certain loci, such as layer II of the anterior cingulate cortex (ACCx-II) and sectors CA3/CA2 of the hippocampus in schizophrenic persons. These two sites receive robust projections from the basolateral amygdala,[13] and based on this observation, it has been postulated that the projections from this region to these two loci may play a pivotal role in the induction of abnormalities. Such changes may be related to the stress response and other emotional reactions mediated through the amygdala.[14,15] Based on the subregional distribution of findings described above, we have developed a "partial" rodent model for neural circuitry abnormalities in postmortem studies of schizophrenia and bipolar disorder.[16] With this model, picrotoxin, an antagonist of the $GABA_A$ receptor, is stereotaxically infused into the BLn.[17] Within 2 hours, a reduction of GABAergic terminals visualized with antibodies against glutamic acid decarboxylase (GAD)65 was observed in sectors CA3 and CA2 but not CA1.[16] This subregional distribution is remarkably similar to that described above for our postmortem studies. We postulated that the changes observed in CA3/CA2 in our postmortem studies could potentially be related to increased glutamatergic activity originating in the BLn.[16]

Identifying Potential Cellular Endophenotypes in Schizophrenia and Bipolar Disorder

Increased glutamatergic activity has been postulated to be present in neural circuits within the brains of schizophrenic persons.[18] Increased excitatory activity emanating from glutamatergic neurons can promote oxidative stress and apoptosis in psychotic disorders.[19] To test the hypothesis that oxidative stress might be present in schizophrenia and possibly also in bipolar disorder, a microarray-based gene expression profiling study was conducted in the hippocampus of normal control subjects, persons with schizophrenia, and persons with bipolar disorder.[20] As shown in Figure 8–1, the results demonstrated a striking difference in the pattern of expression of 24 different genes associated with this signaling pathway in those with schizophrenia and those with bipolar disorder. While the bipolar subjects showed an increased expression of proapoptotic genes, such as FAS ligand and its receptor, tumor necrosis factor alpha, perforin, several caspases, c-myc, and BAK, schizophrenics showed the opposite pattern, i.e., many proapoptotic genes, such as granzyme B and BAX, were either downregulated or showed no change in regulation. Conversely, the antiapoptotic gene, Bcl-2, was found to be upregulated in those with schizophrenia but downregulated in those with bipolar disorder. Additionally, the bipolar subjects showed a highly significant downregulation of several

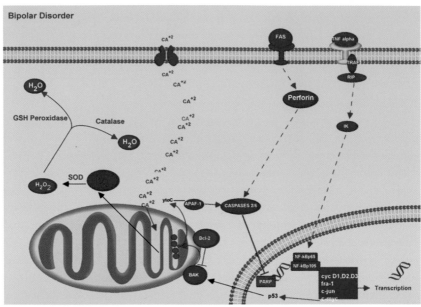

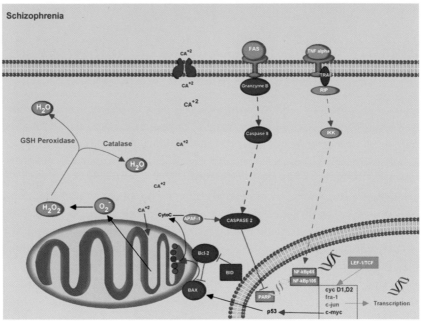

FIGURE 8–1. Schematic diagrams depicting changes in the expression of genes associated with a mitochondrial oxidation, anti-oxidation, and an L-type calcium channel in bipolar disorder *(top)* and schizophrenia *(bottom).*

There are fundamental differences in the regulation of these various genes in the two disorders, with bipolar subjects showing an upregulation (red) of apoptosis, the L-type calcium channel, and mitochondrial oxidation. Taken together with the downregulation of the anti-oxidation enzymes, these changes would mitigate toward dysfunction or even death of hippocampal neurons in this disorder. In schizophrenia, the profile of expression changes is anti-apoptotic. These respective patterns in the two disorders may reflect the presence of uniquely different cellular endophenotypes and reflect differences in the genotype for each.

---

different antioxidation genes, including superoxide dismutase, glutathione peroxidase, glutathione synthase, and catalase, changes that can lead to the accumulation of reactive oxygen species and cellular toxicity.[21] Overall, the results in bipolar subjects were consistent with a previous study in which genes involved in the regulation of the electron transport chain were also found to be markedly downregulated.[22] It is noteworthy that a study of DNA damage in the anterior cingulate cortex demonstrated a marked reduction in schizophrenic but no change in bipolar subjects.[23] Subsequently, a double localization of single-stranded DNA breaks in cells expressing GAD67 messenger RNA demonstrated a significant increase in those with bipolar disorder.[24] Of course, it is important to consider whether neuroleptic drugs may have played a role in these changes. A careful analysis of the regulation of both pro- and antiapoptotic genes in patients with schizophrenia and bipolar disorder who were receiving low versus high doses of these drugs during the year prior to death are not consistent with this possibility.

Taken together, the results described above support the idea that schizophrenia and bipolar disorder involve a common cellular phenotype, one in which dysfunctional GABAergic interneurons contribute to abnormal information processing in the limbic lobe. As suggested by others,[1] the endophenotypes for such cells may nevertheless be quite different in the two different forms of psychotic disorder. It might be concluded then that the mechanisms responsible for the decreased amount of GABAergic activity may be fundamentally different in schizophrenia and bipolar disorder. In bipolar subjects, the gene expression profiling findings clearly point to molecular changes, such as activation of the apoptosis cascade and the L-type calcium channel 1D, but suppression of the antioxidant pathways, that could play a central role in the pathophysiology of this disorder. In schizophrenia, on the other hand, it is unlikely that GABA cell dysfunction involves oxidative mechanisms because similar changes were not observed. Indeed, the regulation of genes associated with apoptosis was suppressed to a large extent. It is important to emphasize, however, that reductions of interneuronal numbers have been found to be reduced in sector CA2 of subjects with both bipolar disorder and schizophrenia.

If the apoptotic cascade were not activated in schizophrenia, why would reduced numbers of GABA cells be found in these patients? One possible explanation for this paradox is that interneurons in the hippocampus of schizophrenic persons are, indeed, being subjected to oxidative stress but only during an earlier phase of the illness. If cells drop out in the schizophrenic subjects, but the apoptotic cascade is subsequently downregulated, the overall number of GABA cells could remain low. If this were the case, it would be difficult to explain the results of a study in which the numerical density of interneurons in CA2 of schizophrenic and bipolar subjects were found to be the same.[25] If apoptosis is indeed killing GABA cells in CA2 of those with bipolar disorder, these cells would be expected to drop out of the neuronal population in that sector. If the regulation of apoptosis genes continues to be upregulated, as it appears to be in bipolar disorder, then one might expect to find that there is an ongoing process of cell loss in these patients as the illness continues. How then can the observation that the number of interneurons is the same in sector CA2 of the bipolar and the schizophrenic subjects be explained? One hypothesis that could account for this apparent discrepancy is that some neurons in the bipolar subjects that undergo apoptosis may have died at an earlier point in time, but others have established a compensation that renders them viable. Alternatively, some cells could be continually replaced through active neurogenesis. In this setting, newly generated cells and cells that are dying would coexist in a relative steady state, such that the overall numbers in CA2 would not appear to be changing. An argument in favor of this hypothesis is that evidence for ongoing apoptosis comes from a study of DNA fragmentation in the anterior cingulate cortex. Specifically, increased DNA damage was observed in GABA cells of the anterior cingulate cortex of bipolar subjects but not schizophrenic subjects.[24] Analogous data for the hippocampus, particularly sector CA2, are not available and it is not necessarily the case that a similar pattern would be observed in this latter subregion.

Conclusions

The above discussion has explored the possibility that molecular endophenotypes for schizophrenia and bipolar disorder may exist at the level of specific circuits, neuronal cell types, and neuronal cell mechanisms. The circuitry inherently present within the limbic lobe, i.e., the anterior cingulate cortex, hippocampus, and basolateral amygdala, together with their reciprocal interconnections, could be part of an endophenotype for each disorder. Presumably, similar substrates may exist in other regions of the brain, such as the dorsolateral prefrontal cortex, that have also been implicated in the pathophysiology of psychotic disorders.[26,27] The GABA cell may be a focus for abnormal expression of many different but functionally interrelated genes.

Despite the apparent similarities between schizophrenia and bipolar disorder observed in our postmortem studies cited above, specific molecular mechanisms appear to be quite different. When not functioning appropriately, alterations of oxidative mechanisms could have the ability to induce dysfunction in bipolar patients and could potentially explain the observation that mood-stabilizing anti-convulsant medications help to stabilize bipolar symptoms.[28,29] For schizophrenic patients, the underlying mechanism for GABA cell dysfunction appears to be fundamentally different. Taken together, these findings are consistent with the hypothesis that a common cellular phenotype (i.e., GABA neuron dysfunction) could theoretically occur through very different cellular mechanisms in two different psychiatric disorders.

It is becoming increasingly clear that our understanding of the nature of endophenotypes for psychotic disorders will require a careful delineation of brain regions, circuits, neuronal subtypes, and the associated cellular mechanisms that underlie the clinical manifestations of these illnesses. In clinical investigations, complex markers, such as temporal stability of antisaccades,[30] event-related potentials,[31] and working memory,[32] have also been used to distinguish endophenotypes for schizophrenia versus bipolar disorder. As with postmortem studies in which a notable downregulation of GAD67 expression has been observed in both diagnostic groups,[26,33] significant similarities in markers, such as working memory, have also been observed in studies of schizophrenia and bipolar disorder.[32] Such endophenotypic overlap may well indicate the presence of common environmental influences occurring in such individuals with the two disorders. Nevertheless, the fact that there now appear to be discrete differences in the pattern of gene expression in the hippocampus of schizophrenic and bipolar subjects makes it increasingly likely that the endophenotypes for these two disorders may also include unique cellular and molecular substrates specific to each disorder. An understanding of what constitutes a brain endophenotype requires that we learn more about the ways in which candidate neurons are being regulated and influencing brain regions, and how, in turn, neurons comprising complex circuits may or may not respond to either intrinsic or extrinsic inputs within larger circuits. Ultimately, neurobiological information of this type will eventually provide a precise understanding of differences in the cellular and molecular regulation of neurons within affected circuits, and will bring us closer to understanding the underlying genotype for each disorder.

The fact that there are similarities in the clinical phenotype for schizophrenia and bipolar disorder suggests that the respective endophenotypes may also show areas of overlap with respect to the circuitry involved and the nature of the cellular and molecular changes present. Contrariwise, the fact that these two disorders show prominent differences in their clinical phenotypes implies that other aspects of limbic lobe circuitry and GABA cell integration may show abnormalities that are unique to each disorder. The data presented above provide support for this hypothesis. Having similarities and differences in clinical phenotype and, by inference, endophenotype makes the process of defining the respective neural substrates quite difficult and time consuming. Toward this end, the use of postmortem tissues in combination with molecular strategies, such as gene expression profiling and genome-wide association studies, will be a critical element in the overall strategy to use two-factor modeling to uncover heritable and environmental components of a complex psychiatric endophenotype.

References

1. Gottesman II, Gould TD. The endophenotype concept in psychiatry: etymology and strategic intentions. Am J Psychiatry. 2003;160:636–645.
2. Kety SS, Rosenthal D, Wender PH, Schulsinger F, Jacobsen B. Mental illness in the biological and adoptive families of adopted individuals who have become schizophrenic. Behav Genet. 1976;6:219–225.
3. Hasler G, Drevets WC, Gould TD, Gottesman II, Manji HK. Toward constructing an endophenotype strategy for bipolar disorders. Biol Psychiatry. 2006;60:93–105.
4. Leonard S, Adams C, Breese CR, et al. Nicotinic receptor function in schizophrenia. Schizophr Bull. 1996;22:431–445.
5. Schadt EE, Sachs A, Friend S. Embracing complexity, inching closer to reality. Sci STKE. 2005;(295):pe40.
6. Simpson MD, Slater P, Deakin JF, Royston MC, Skan WJ. Reduced GABA uptake sites in the temporal lobe in schizophrenia. Neurosci Lett. 1989;107:211–215.
7. Heckers S, Heinsen H, Heinsen YC, Beckmann H. Limbic structures and lateral ventricle in schizophrenia. A quantitative postmortem study. [see comments]. Arch Gen Psychiatry. 1990;47:1016–1022.
8. Reynolds GP, Czudek C, Andrews HB. Deficit and hemispheric asymmetry of GABA uptake sites in the hippocampus in schizophrenia. Biol Psychiatry. 1990;27:1038–1044.
9. Reynolds GP. The amygdala and the neurochemistry of schizophrenia. In: Aggleton JP, ed. The Amygdala. New York: Wiley-Liss; 1992.
10. Longson D, Deakin JF, Benes FM. Increased density of entorhinal glutamate-immunoreactive vertical fibers in schizophrenia. J Neural Transm. 1996;103:503–507.
11. Simpson MD, Slater P, Deakin JF. Comparison of glutamate and gamma-aminobutyric acid uptake binding sites in frontal and temporal lobes in schizophrenia. Biol Psychiatry. 1998;44:423–427.
12. Benes FM. Emerging principles of altered neural circuitry in schizophrenia. Brain Res Rev. 2000;31:251–269.
13. Benes FM, Berretta S. Amygdalo-entorhinal inputs to the hippocampal formation in relation to schizophrenia. Ann NY Acad Sci. 2000;911:293–304.
14. LeDoux JE. Emotion circuits in the brain. Annu Rev Neurosci. 2000;23:155–184.
15. Antoniadis EA, McDonald RJ. Amygdala, hippocampus and discriminative fear conditioning to context. Behav Brain Res. 2000;108:1–19.

16. Berretta S, Munno DW, Benes FM. Amygdalar activation alters the hippocampal GABA system: "partial" modelling for postmortem changes in schizophrenia. J Comp Neurol. 2001;431:129–138.

17. Benes FM, Berretta S. Amygdalo-entorhinal inputs to the hippocampal formation in relation to schizophrenia. Ann NY Acad Sci. 2000;911:293–304.

18. Benes FM, Sorensen I, Vincent SL, Bird ED, Sathi M. Increased density of glutamate-immunoreactive vertical processes in superficial laminae in cingulate cortex of schizophrenic brain. Cereb Cortex. 1992;2:503–512.

19. Coyle JT, Puttfarcken P. Oxidative stress, glutamate, and neurodegenerative disorders [review]. Science. 1993;262:689–695.

20. Benes FM, Matzilevich D, Burke RE, Walsh J. The expression of proapoptosis genes is increased in bipolar disorder, but not in schizophrenia. Mol Psychiatry. 2006;11:241–251.

21. Rego AC, Monteiro NM, Silva AP, Gil J, Malva JO, Oliveira CR. Mitochondrial apoptotic cell death and moderate superoxide generation upon selective activation of non-desensitizing AMPA receptors in hippocampal cultures. J Neurochem. 2003;86:792–804.

22. Konradi C, Eaton M, MacDonald ML, Walsh J, Benes FM, Heckers S. Molecular evidence for mitochondrial dysfunction in bipolar disorder. Arch Gen Psychiatry. 2004;61:300–308.

23. Benes FM, Walsh J, Bhattacharyya S, Sheth A, Berretta S. DNA fragmentation decreased in schizophrenia but not bipolar disorder. Arch Gen Psychiatry. 2003;60:359–364.

24. Buttner N, Bhattacharyya S, Walsh JP, Benes FM. DNA fragmentation is increased in non-GABAeregic neurons in bipolar disorder. Schizophr Res. 2007;93:33–41.

25. Benes FM, Kwok EW, Vincent SL, Todtenkopf MS. A reduction of nonpyramidal cells in sector CA2 of schizophrenics and manic depressives. Biol Psychiatry. 1998;44:88–97.

26. Guidotti A, Auta J, Davis JM, et al. Decrease in reelin and glutamic acid decarboxylase 67 (GAD67) expression in schizophrenia and bipolar disorder: a postmortem brain study. Arch Gen Psychiatry. 2000;57:1061–1069.

27. Akbarian S, Kim JJ, Potkin SG, et al. Gene expression for glutamic acid decarboxylase is reduced without loss of neurons in prefrontal cortex of schizophrenics. Arch Gen Psychiatry. 1995;52:258–266.

28. Li X, Bijur GN, Jope RS. Glycogen synthase kinase-3beta, mood stabilizers, and neuroprotection. Bipolar Disord. 2002;4:137–144.

29. Gould TD, Chen G, Manji HK. In vivo evidence in the brain for lithium inhibition of glycogen synthase kinase-3. Neuropsychopharmacology. 2004;29:32–38.

30. Gooding DC, Iacono WG, Katsanis J, Beiser M, Grove WM. Temporal stability of saccadic task performance in schizophrenia and bipolar patients. Psychol Med. 2004;34:921–932.

31. Hall MH, Rijsdijk F, Kalidindi S, et al. Genetic overlap between bipolar illness and event-related potentials. Psychol Med. 2007;37:667–678.

32. Szoke A, Schurhoff F, Golmard JL, et al. Familial resemblance for executive functions in families of schizophrenic and bipolar patients. Psychiatry Res. 2006;144:131–138.

33. Woo TU, et al. Density of glutamic acid decarboxylase 67 messenger RNA-containing neurons that express the N-methyl-D-aspartate receptor subunit NR2A in the anterior cingulate cortex in schizophrenia and bipolar disorder. Arch Gen Psychiatry. 2004;61:649–657.

9

DECONSTRUCTING PSYCHOSIS WITH HUMAN BRAIN IMAGING

Raquel E. Gur, M.D., Ph.D.
Matcheri S. Keshavan, M.D.
Stephen M. Lawrie, M.D., FRCPsych

Advances in neuroimaging technologies have created both opportunities and challenges in the study of psychosis. Eager to obtain a "window to the mind," neuroimaging has been embraced by investigators applying diverse methods to examine brain structure and function in psychiatric disorders. With progress in quantitative computational anatomy methodologies, we are at the threshold of an exciting era in psychiatric research that can capitalize on the ability to study the living brain with refined approaches both for hypothesis testing and for exploration. In vivo measurement is afforded by magnetic resonance imaging (MRI) examining neuroanatomy through structural MRI (sMRI), connectivity through diffusion tensor imaging (DTI), and neurochemistry through magnetic resonance spectroscopy (MRS). Magnetic resonance also enables examination of brain physiology using functional MRI (fMRI)

Reprinted with permission from Gur RE, Keshavan MS, Lawrie SM. "Deconstructing Psychosis With Human Brain Imaging." *Schizophrenia Bulletin* 2007; 33: 921–931.

This report was supported by the following grants: MH64045 and MH60722 (Gur), MH64023 and MH45156 (Keshavan), Dr. Mortimer and Theresa Sackler Foundation (Lawrie).

methods. Other functional neuroimaging methods include positron emission tomography (PET), which enables measurement of local cerebral glucose metabolism, blood flow, and receptor function. Single-photon computed emission tomography (SPECT) can also be used to measure cerebral perfusion and receptor function.

The diversity and complementarity of neuroimaging methods can place them in a crucial position for integrative translational research. Neuroimaging can intersect basic and clinical efforts in elucidating the underlying processes of complex psychotic disorders. By supplying data obtained on patients, neuroimaging has a firm hold on the clinical phenotype, and by informing on brain systems, it can link to molecular substrates. Furthermore, combining neuroimaging with genetic strategies can yield a powerful methodology with unprecedented potential for novel treatments (Figure 9–1). The challenge we face is making this happen by mobilizing the increasing array of procedures and measures relevant to clinically important questions such as diagnosis, course of illness, and outcome.

After three decades of neuroimaging research, is the technology informative to efforts to deconstruct psychosis? Based on brain imaging studies can we examine a patient with first-episode psychosis and determine with some confidence whether schizophrenia or bipolar disorder is on the horizon? Might we even be able to use imaging as an early diagnostic aid in those at genetic or symptomatic high risk?

The research agenda in neuroimaging and psychosis has not been geared from the outset to be clinically relevant in differential diagnosis. Rather, most studies in psychosis have focused on one disorder with the explicit primary goal of understanding its specific pathophysiology. An implicit secondary goal has been to improve diagnosis and clinical management. When imaging, commonly structural, has been applied clinically as part of the workup of a psychotic patient, the purpose has been to rule out a space-occupying lesion or developmental malformation that may potentially cause the psychosis. Although incidental findings have been reported in MRI studies of even healthy people[1] and patients who present with psychosis,[2] such findings are infrequent and commonly asymptomatic. This is not to say that obtaining a scan is of no value where an organic psychosis is suspected; in a recent analysis of 253 adult psychiatric patients who underwent a clinical MRI, 38 (15%) had some form of treatment modification as a result of the neuroimaging findings, and in 6 patients a medical condition was identified as a result of the MRI.[3] However, in the absence of quantitative analysis, routine brain imaging cannot aid in the differential diagnosis of psychosis without considering the clinical presentation.[4] Thus far, studies using imaging techniques to determine prognosis or treatment response have not generated sufficiently replicated findings. There are, however, encouraging results from several studies evaluating these technologies as possible predictors of diagnosis.

Most neuroimaging studies have been conducted in schizophrenia. A PubMed search in October 2006 showed 490 citations for "schizophrenia and neuroimaging" and only 134 for "bipolar and neuroimaging." Only 31 studies are cited for

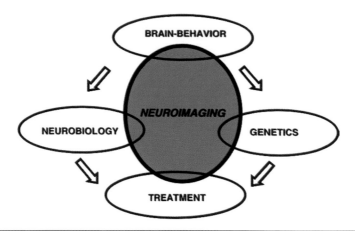

FIGURE 9–1. A schematic representation of the central role of neuroimaging intersecting between basic science and clinical applications.

the conjunctive "schizophrenia and bipolar and neuroimaging" query. Few prospective studies contain the information that would permit comparison between patients with schizophrenia and those with bipolar illness. Inconsistent findings within disorders have often led to controversy and have been attributed to disease heterogeneity. Over the past decade, advances in quantitative techniques have established some firm findings about schizophrenia and related disorders. As importantly, these techniques have also highlighted areas where further study is required and where methodological practices need to be improved.

This chapter will briefly highlight the knowledge we have gained about psychosis using brain imaging methods by emphasizing the results from consistently replicated studies, systematic reviews, and meta-analyses of the relevant literature. We shall consider structural imaging (sMRI, DTI), neurochemical imaging (MRS, receptor studies), and functional imaging techniques in patients with schizophrenia and the affective psychoses, including studies of at-risk populations. The latter enable integration of genetic and neuroimaging paradigms in our efforts to elucidate neurobiological mechanisms that underlie these disorders that may guide treatments.

Structural Magnetic Resonance Imaging and Diffusion Tensor Imaging

SMRI STUDIES OF PATIENTS

An extensive literature, presented in reviews[4–6] and meta-analyses,[7–11] documents consistent morphometric differences between patients with schizophrenia and healthy people. There is whole-brain volume reduction of about 3% in patients, particularly in gray matter,[7,8] and a concomitant increase in cerebrospinal fluid (CSF). Volume reductions have been most notable in frontotemporal regions. Medial temporal lobe (MTL) structures and, particularly, the hippocampus and amygdala are reduced by a greater amount than the whole brain.[6,10] This is also probably true of the prefrontal cortex (PFC) and other parts of the temporal lobe, particularly the superior temporal gyrus (STG).[5,8] There is evidence that the thalamus is likewise reduced in volume to a greater extent than the whole brain.[11] The size of the corpus callosum, a white matter fiber bundle, is reduced to a roughly similar extent as the whole brain.[9]

The region of interest (ROI) analytic approach initially applied has been replaced by automated methods for regional parcellation and voxel-based morphometry that can efficiently yield information on the entire brain, permitting validation of reported findings and new discovery of other affected regions. Based on morphological parameters, it is possible to apply high-dimensional nonlinear pattern classification techniques to quantify the degree of separation of patients with schizophrenia and healthy control subjects. Such procedures enable testing the potential of sMRI as an aid to diagnosis. In a recent study of patients with schizophrenia and healthy control subjects, such a procedure demonstrated average classification accuracy of 82% for women and 85% for men.[12] While such automated methods are promising, further investigation is needed, and we cannot yet rely solely upon such approaches.

Whole-brain size reductions observed in schizophrenia have been demonstrated to have "concurrent validity" by quantitative review of postmortem studies.[13] A review of computational voxel-based morphometry studies highlighted that they consistently find gray matter density reductions in MTLs and the STG.[14] Furthermore, there are replicated associations between STG volumes and positive symptoms and between MTL reductions and memory impairment.[6,15,16] Figure 9–2 illustrates application of deformation-based morphometry to compare a sample of patients with schizophrenia with healthy control subjects.[12]

These abnormalities are unlikely to be confounded by factors such as antipsychotic medication or substance abuse. Most MRI studies that examined the specific ROIs, highlighted above, also evaluated possible relationships with antipsychotic medication status or dosages and very rarely find any—with the exception of some parts of the basal ganglia. In particular, increases of up to 20% in the volume of the globus pallidus are regularly related to first-generation (typical) antipsychotic medication dosage.[8] A review examining the effect of typical antipsychotics on brain structure revealed basal ganglia volume increases and cortical gray matter decreases, detectable even after a 12-week treatment period.[17] However, most studies have involved indirect and nonrandomized comparisons in analyses that seemingly seek to establish that the second-generation (atypical) antipsychotics have beneficial effects on neuroanatomy. There are no consistently replicated accounts of particular drugs having beneficial effects in specific brain re-

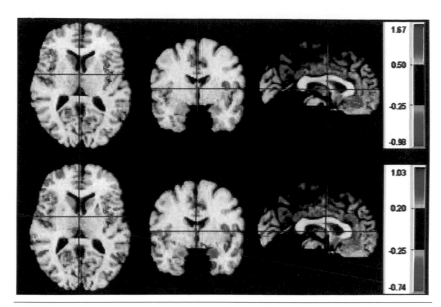

FIGURE 9–2. Effect sizes of control/patient group difference, calculated separately for neuroleptic-naive *(top)* and treated patients with schizophrenia *(bottom)*.

The spatial patterns are similar, except that treated patients display generally stronger effect sizes. *Blue* means that the respective structures were relatively larger in patients than in healthy control subjects. Thus, treated patients showed a pronounced increase in basal ganglia volumes.

Source. Reprinted with permission from Davatzikos et al.[12] Copyright (2005) American Medical Association. All rights reserved.

gions. Because patients with psychosis may have comorbid substance abuse, the possible effects of such substances should also be considered. The effects of alcohol abuse on the brain are usually generalized, or show a PFC rather than temporal lobe bias, and the abnormalities in schizophrenia noted above are present in patients with no history of alcohol abuse. It is unclear if cannabis has any effects on brain structure, and other substances are used too infrequently to be likely confounders.

More pertinent limitations of this literature are highlighted in a recent review of sMRI in first-episode schizophrenia studies that confirms only a reduction in the volumes of the whole brain and of the hippocampus.[18] This raises the clear need for further studies of recent-onset patients to determine if other abnormalities are evident at that time or if they are progressive;[19] although it will clearly be very difficult, if not impossible, to distinguish the effects of illness duration from the effects of ongoing antipsychotic treatment.

Notably, similar findings, at least concerning the whole brain and hippocampus, are evident in dementia. The cognitive deficits in schizophrenia and its early characterization as dementia praecox buttress that similar brain systems may be affected, with an underlying different neuropathology and decades apart. Of more direct clinical concern, as the structural neuroimaging literature in bipolar disorder and depression accrues, it seems that the neuroanatomy of affective disorder is qualitatively similar to that in schizophrenia but merely less marked in quantitative terms. At present, the only disease-specific finding is that patients with bipolar disorder may not have whole-brain volume reduction that is evident in schizophrenia, [20–23] may not show volume reductions in amygdala, and may even show volume increases in amygdala at particular stages of the illness.[23] It is now clear that the hippocampus is reduced in volume even in depression.[24,25] These hippocampal reductions may be related to the number of depressive episodes and may even be more marked in patients with severe depression than in the general population of patients with schizophrenia. Finally, there are consistent reports and meta-analyses of an increased frequency of signal hyperintensities in affective disorder[22–27] that may be specific but of uncertain pathologenesis.

There have been too few direct comparisons of patients with schizophrenia and bipolar disorder, let alone other psychoses, to evaluate neuroanatomical differences among the disorders. These studies have relatively small samples and few have addressed changes over time—the basis on which the disorders were originally separated. A useful strategy that can address the issue of diagnostic specificity is the study of patients with first-episode psychosis who are followed longitudinally. Once the diagnosis is established, intake sMRI measures are examined for possible differences among groups.[28–32] The available reports are inconsistent. For example, left prefrontal gray matter volume reduction was noted in first-episode schizophrenia and not in affective psychosis.[28] However, in male adolescents, increased CSF and reduced gray matter volumes in the frontal lobes did not distinguish those who developed schizophrenia from those who did not.[31] Such studies are important because they enable testing the hypothesis that there is more progression of abnormalities in those with first-episode psychosis who go on to develop schizophrenia as compared with affective disorder, but this key question would be much more practicably and quickly addressed in multicenter than single-center studies.

There is a relative lack of studies in the affective disorders examining the associations of sMRI findings to clinical and neurobehavioral features. In schizophrenia, there are demonstrated associations between memory difficulties and positive psychotic symptoms and the size of the hippocampus, the STG, and the temporal lobe in general and between executive function, negative symptoms, and PFC measures,[6,15,16] but these relationships have not been documented in bipolar disorder.

DIFFUSION TENSOR IMAGING

DTI examines white matter integrity and is a more recent addition to structural measures (Figure 9–3). As might be expected with such a rapidly developing technology, there are some replicated findings in the schizophrenia literature, but it has

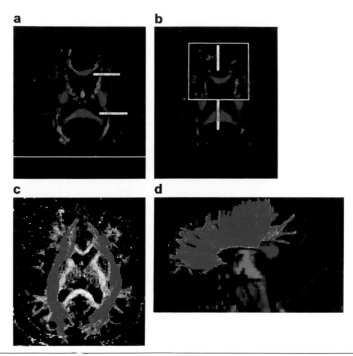

FIGURE 9–3. Illustration of DTI measures showing fractional anisotropy *(a, b)*, with delineation of specific regions of interest, corresponding white matter tracts can be visualized showing front back *(c)* and left-right callosal connectivity *(d)*.

Source. Courtesy of R. Verma, University of Pennsylvania.

been particularly hampered by the wide array of different approaches both to acquire the data and to analyze them.[33] With the development of tractography techniques, a common approach by the imaging community could facilitate progress. Although gray matter volume deficits are more marked than white matter abnormalities in schizophrenia, reduced anisotropy (a measure of directionality of flow of water molecules in axons, thereby an index of white matter integrity) is observed with DTI in many brain regions. This finding suggests that white matter structure may be disorganized in schizophrenia rather than reduced in size.[33] One major appeal of DTI is that it can directly test the prevailing view of schizophrenia (and psychosis in general) as a disconnection disorder.

STUDIES OF RELATIVES AND OTHERS "AT RISK"

sMRI studies of the MTL have been the focus of most attention in people at risk. Early ROI studies tended to examine the amygdala and hippocampus together and consistently found reductions in relatives compared with control subjects, but most relatives did not have volume reductions to pathological levels.[15,34] The balance of the evidence was for hippocampal differences in particular, although there were some notable and quite large negative studies. A comprehensive review concluded that reduced hippocampi were likely to be a vulnerability marker for schizophrenia.[15] This view has recently been supported by a systematic review and meta-analysis of studies of relatives that finds hippocampal reductions in relatives, with an effect size of about 0.3, and additional differences between relatives and patients.[35]

Despite the small number of studies, there are already replicated computational voxel-based morphometry studies in the relatives of patients with schizophrenia versus bipolar disorder. Both Job et al.[36] and Diwadkar et al.[37] found reduced gray matter in PFC in relatives at high risk for schizophrenia. Similarly, both McIntosh et al.[38] and McDonald et al.[39] have reported reductions in gray matter density in prefrontal regions and thalamus in schizophrenia as distinct from no reductions in gray matter in these regions in bipolar disorder. Reductions in the thalamus have been reported as a measure of genetic liability to psychosis in general.[39,40]

The implication of such findings is that there are dissociable state- and trait-imaging markers of psychosis. Therefore, vulnerability markers may predict schizophrenia before clinical presentation, expecting further volume reduction near the onset of psychosis. The two main studies to have addressed these issues to date are the Edinburgh High-Risk Study (EHRS) and the study conducted in the Personal Assessment and Crisis Evaluation Clinic in Melbourne, Australia. These pioneering studies have examined large populations of people at risk, for genetic or clinical reasons, over almost 10 years. A total of five articles have been published by these two research groups concerning the possible predictive utility of a reduced hippocampal volume, and even different reports from the same study are conflicting. Thus, it seems that any predictive effect is inconsistent and at most weak.[41–45] More encouragingly, both groups have also evaluated changes in brain structure over time and reported complementary results. Pantelis et al.[42] demonstrated reductions in gray matter in the left parahippocampal and fusiform gyri, as well as other regions in frontal and left cerebellar cortex, over approximately a year in 11 people as they developed a diagnosis of psychosis, usually schizophrenia. Job et al.[43] revealed reductions in gray matter density in left (para) hippocampal uncus, fusiform gyrus, and right cerebellar cortex in 8 individuals at high risk, for familial reasons, who developed schizophrenia on average 2.5 years after the first of two scans, obtained approximately 18 months apart. This replication suggests reductions in temporal lobe structure around the time of transition to diagnosis of psychosis and, to some extent, predating the conversion. The EHRS in particular makes it clear that such changes may occur years prior to diagnosis and cannot be attributable to medication because none of the participants were medicated until after their second scan and their diagnosis was established.

The Edinburgh group has gone a step further and evaluated the diagnostic properties of these reductions in gray matter density as a possible "early diagnostic test," by comparing the 8 subjects who had two scans and developed schizophrenia with either 10 patients with similar psychotic symptoms at the time of scanning who did not go on to have schizophrenia or 57 high-risk subjects who had two scans regardless of whether or not they had symptoms. In both cases, temporal lobe volume reductions showed very promising diagnostic properties, with positive predictive values (PPVs) of around 70% for these regional reductions individually and about 80% in combination.[46] These PPVs can be contrasted with much lower values for psychotic symptoms and behavioral measures. In the high-risk study, approximately 12.5% of those "at risk" developed schizophrenia, as did (only) 25% of those with psychotic symptoms, about 30% of those scoring poorly on the Rey Auditory Verbal Learning Test, and approximately 50% of those scoring above the cutoff on schizotypy measures.[44] Structural imaging clearly adds clinical value here, but there are important questions about the practicality of using such an approach in clinical practice, and early diagnosis would only be justified if an intervention was available for such patients.

A major limitation is the very small sample sizes in these studies. Replication with larger samples is needed and can best be achieved in multicenter collaborations. The standardization of imaging techniques and approaches to analysis is essential for deriving a "human brain map" with detailed information about relevant changes in brain structure during the normal range of neurodevelopment. Such extensive information might be required before significant progress can be made in applying structural imaging techniques to clinical issues in psychosis.

Neurochemical Imaging

MAGNETIC RESONANCE SPECTROSCOPY

MRS provides a noninvasive tool to investigate metabolites in the living human brain. Being safe, this technique allows investigation of the effects of the illness course as well as the medications on these metabolites. Much MRS work has focused on investigating phosphorus (^{31}P-MRS) and proton-containing metabolites (^{1}H-MRS).[47,48]

Proton MRS metabolites include *N*-acetyl aspartate (NAA), creatine, choline, myoinositol, glutamine, glutamate, glutathione, and γ-aminobutyric acid (GABA). NAA is mainly synthesized in neurons and is therefore regarded as a putative marker for neuronal loss or dysfunction.[49,50] However, NAA levels may also reflect the integrity of glial cells.[51] NAA is also important for membrane phospholipid and mitochondrial metabolism.[52,53]

A reduction in NAA peaks is found in most studies of patients with chronic schizophrenia. Such deficits encompass several brain regions, notably hippocampus and frontal cortex. A recent systematic review and meta-analysis of 64 published studies involving 1,209 schizophrenia patients and 1,256 control subjects suggested consistent evidence of NAA reductions in the frontal lobes and the hippocampus.[54] NAA reductions appear to be associated with cortical atrophy, cognitive impairment, and negative symptoms.[48] Furthermore, NAA reductions have been correlated with increased illness duration,[55] supporting the possibility of a progressive impairment of neuronal integrity as the illness unfolds.

NAA reductions are established and clinically used in studies of several neurological disorders, including stroke and multiple sclerosis. Among psychiatric disorders, euthymic bipolar patients have decreases in NAA in frontal lobe structures and hippocampus, reported in a review of 22 studies involving 328 adult bipolar and 349 control subjects.[56] On the other hand, a systematic review and meta-analysis of major depressive disorder (MDD) by the same authors indicated increased choline-containing metabolites in the basal ganglia but no alteration of NAA.[57] The diagnostic specificity of NAA reduction remains to be further clarified.

NAA reductions are present in first-degree relatives who are at genetic high risk (GHR) for schizophrenia, although the results are more variable than in patients. Nonpsychotic relatives of schizophrenia patients showed NAA/choline ratio reductions in the anterior cingulate.[34,58] By contrast, Tibbo et al.[59] observed elevated glutamatergic metabolites but no other metabolite alterations in high-risk offspring of schizophrenia patients in a 3T MRS study. Jessen et al.[60] used proton MRS to examine neurochemical characteristics of the brain in people deemed clinically at high risk (CHR) for schizophrenia (the prodromal state, defined by the presence of subthreshold psychotic-like symptoms). They observed that reduced NAA/choline ratios in the anterior cingulate predicted psychosis during longitudinal follow-up. Wood et al.[61] reported increased NAA/creatine ratios in the dorsolateral prefrontal cortex in CHR subjects; this finding did not predict those who "converted" to schizophrenia during follow-up. Collectively, these observations suggest that alterations of NAA in prefrontal structures may represent a vulnerability indicator for schizophrenia in GHR subjects and even less consistently in CHR subjects. More data are needed to replicate these observations if they are to be of any value as clinically useful predictive markers for schizophrenia.

^{31}P-MRS investigations in drug-naive first-episode psychosis patients suggest increased membrane breakdown at the onset of psychosis,[62–65] and in most studies, there appears to be reduced membrane generation in early and chronic schizophrenia. Cell membrane changes occur prominently during cell generation and synaptogenesis, but also during cell degenerative processes such as apoptotic elimination of dendrites and axons (pruning) and cell death. Cell membrane alterations of patients with schizophrenia are also well documented in peripheral and postmortem brain tissue at different stages of the disorder (for review see Berger et al.[66]). Such findings may reflect a reduction in neurons, glia, or synapses in schizophrenia. Studies of adolescent offspring at increased genetic risk for schizophrenia show membrane alterations similar to those observed in patients with early schizophrenia;[67] these changes are more pronounced in the at-risk adolescents who have already begun to manifest psychopathology.[68]

Interestingly, patients with manic psychosis appear to have an increase in membrane precursors,[69] which may reflect a compensatory increase in cell generation or synaptogenesis during manic exacerbation of psychotic disorders. This suggests that there might be some measure of diagnostic specificity for ^{31}P-MRS changes, but the number of studies in bipolar patients and other psychiatric disorders is too small to have confident application of these findings as clinical markers for diagnosis.

NEURORECEPTOR STUDIES

PET and SPECT provide an important avenue to examine in vivo neurochemistry. The investigation of receptor function with PET followed progress with in vitro binding measurements and autoradiography. Earlier ligand studies in schizophrenia have examined primarily dopamine (DA) receptor properties and particularly D_2. The application of D_2 receptor PET studies to neuroleptic-naive patients yielded initially somewhat inconsistent results; data from Johns Hopkins investigators showed increased occupancy with $[^{11}C]$-*N*-methylspiperone,[70] but Karolinska investigators using $[^{11}C]$-raclopride did not.[71] These discrepancies in the literature might be related to several factors, such as differences in patient population, ligands used, and modeling methods.[72] The emphasis in studying neuroleptic-naive patients in a limited number of settings that can apply the technology resulted in relatively small samples with commonly less than 20 patients per study. However, an early systematic review of 17 postmortem and PET studies found a large effect size of almost 1.5,[73] accompanied by increases in both D_2 receptor density and affinity. Several comprehensive reviews have come to the same conclusion.[74,75]

A consistent literature has emerged indicating increased presynaptic dopaminergic turnover in schizophrenia. Such studies measured striatal fluorodopa uptake as an index of increased dopa decarboxylase activity and greater presynaptic DA turnover in the striatum. Increased activity of DA neurons in the striatum appears to be associated with clinical status and is more evident during acute exacerbations and presence of positive symptoms.[75] Notably, such effects are consistent with studies of neuropharmacological stimulants, such as amphetamine, and cannot be attributed to antipsychotic medication because, approximately, half the studies have been conducted in medication-free, including neuroleptic-naive, patients.

Increased striatal DA, most evident in patients with active psychotic symptoms, has been related to the positive symptoms of schizophrenia. More recently, neuroreceptor studies have related DA function to cognitive processes in schizophrenia. Cortical DA transmission via D_1 receptors may play a role in impaired working memory and negative symptoms,[76] whereas striatal DA activity via D_2 receptors may modulate response inhibition, temporal organization, and motor performance.[77]

Most neuroreceptor studies have been conducted in patients with schizophrenia, and it is unclear if the relation between striatal DA function and psychosis is unique to schizophrenia or is evident in other disorders with psychotic features. Recent PET studies in bipolar disorder have examined different systems implicated in the pathophysiology of the disorder including serotonin transporter binding[78] and the muscarinic receptor.[79] Thus, there is insufficient knowledge to determine whether receptor neuroimaging can be helpful in differentiating among psychotic disorders.

Receptor imaging by PET and SPECT allows investigation of in vivo targets for antipsychotic drug action.[80] It is now known that extrapyramidal (parkinsonian) side effects of first-generation antipsychotic drugs result from high striatal DA D_2 receptor blockade (~75%), while second-generation antipsychotic drugs produce therapeutic benefit in relation to modest and transient striatal D_2 receptor occupancy levels (~65%). These neuroimaging observations point to a rationale for the use of relatively low doses of first-generation antipsychotics and equivalent doses of second-generation antipsychotics,[81] although use of neuroimaging to determine dosage ranges in a given patient is far from practical. Neuroreceptor PET/SPECT studies are valuable research tools that can help examine compounds that may regulate or stabilize DA as well as nondopaminergic pathways such as serotonin, glutamate, and GABA that may offer promising targets for drug development.

Functional Imaging

STUDIES OF PATIENTS

The functional imaging literature in schizophrenia has evolved from PET studies measuring glucose metabolism and blood flow to fMRI studies with activation paradigms. Diverse neurobehavioral probes have been applied in activation paradigms, designed to elucidate the underlying brain circuitry. Tasks applied have evaluated executive function such as attention, abstraction, and working memory as well as declarative and procedural memory, language, spatial, sensorimotor, and emotion processing. The breadth of approaches has precluded the establishment of a functional imaging phenotype of schizophrenia. Nonetheless, there is an emerging consistency of findings.[82]

The early emphasis on "hypofrontality" in schizophrenia has been refined. A review of the PET literature found 21 resting studies with an overall effect size of 0.64 and 9 activation studies with an overall effect size of 1.13.[83] A more recent review of PET and SPECT studies examined 47 reports with relative resting measures of cerebral activity, 29 with absolute resting baseline measures, and 14 activation paradigms. Studies with neurobehavioral probes included similar numbers of those using the Wisconsin Card Sort Test, the Continuous Performance Task, and a variety of other probes. While some similarity in the pattern of brain activity was observed across experiments, there was substantial heterogeneity.[84] A potential strength in activation studies is the ability to relate the extent of activation to performance obtained "on line." However, relative underactivation in patients who have difficulties performing a task may reflect a deficit in underlying processes related to that task or lack of engagement.[84,85] Notably, PET and fMRI studies that attempted to correct for patients'

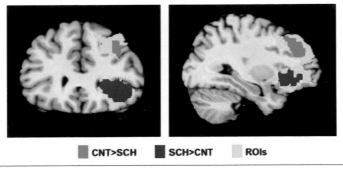

CNT>SCH   **SCH>CNT**   ROIs

FIGURE 9–4.   An fMRI word-encoding study showing connectivity differences between patients with schizophrenia and healthy control subjects in left superior temporal gyrus (STG) to dorsolateral prefrontal cortex (DLPFC) and to ventrolateral prefrontal cortex (VLPFC).

A region of DLPFC shows greater connectivity with STG in controls, while a region in VLPFC shows greater connectivity with STG in patients.

CNT = control subject; ROIs = regions of interest; SCH = patient with schizophrenia.

Source.   Reprinted with permission from Wolf et al.[99] Copyright (2007) Elsevier.

impairment, by balancing performance of patients and healthy control subjects, often found no hypofrontality or even hyperfrontality.[14] In two recent systematic reviews, however, 12 N-back (working memory) fMRI studies and 18 episodic memory studies with PET or fMRI found "hypofrontality" in dorsolateral and inferolateral PFC, respectively.[86,87] Glahn et al.[87] also reported hyperfrontality in medial areas including (dorsal) anterior cingulate. Antipsychotic medication is likely to normalize performance on these tasks and hypofrontality.[88] While the majority of studies were conducted in patients with schizophrenia, reduced or increased frontal lobe activity is also evident in bipolar disorder,[21,22] but direct comparisons of the groups are rare.[89]

Regarding the temporal lobe, an early review found fairly consistent evidence of increased temporal lobe activity in 13 SPECT studies and 6 PET studies.[90] These increases were cortical, but Achim and Lepage[86] recently reported bilateral reductions in perfusion in the MTLs. Perhaps a hypothesis that will incorporate these findings will evaluate the interaction between laterality and frontality. For example, lateral cortex hypofrontality and hypertemporality may interact with a mirror image in medial hyperfrontality-hypotemporality.

Such a synthesis of the available literature for lateral cortical regions is certainly in keeping with early and contemporary accounts of the disconnectivity hypothesis of schizophrenia and replicated findings of reduced frontotemporal and frontoparietal functional connectivity.[91,92] PET, SPECT, and fMRI studies (Figure 9–4) of disconnectivity are also supported by accounts of reduced coherence and gamma asynchrony with electroencephalography and magnetoencephalography in schizophrenia.[93,94] Where medial regions have been invoked in such systems, it has usually been in terms of medial frontal regions modulating lateral frontotemporal interactions. There is, as yet, no systematic review of this literature and no generally adopted approach to acquiring and processing data for functional and effective connectivity analyses. Establishing such a framework must be another priority for the imaging community.

STUDIES IN RELATIVES AND CLINICAL UTILITIES

Functional imaging studies in family members of patients with schizophrenia are limited. There are fewer than 10 perfusion studies and fewer still reports of disconnectivity. There are approximately equal numbers of accounts of hypofrontality, no significant perfusion deficits, and hyperfrontality under different conditions.[95] More obviously consistent are replicated accounts of PFC disconnectivity.[96–99]

Comparative studies of diagnostic specificity are again few. The possibilities of using functional imaging, and particularly ligand binding, to predict treatment response and prognosis have also been understudied, with few replicated results. In a preliminary "proof of concept" study from the EHRS, fMRI could indeed predict the later development of schizophrenia—but this was in a post hoc analysis of only four patients.[98]

FUNCTIONAL IMAGING IN RELATION TO TREATMENT

Several studies have examined changes in abnormal brain function in relation to antipsychotic medications. Davis et al.[88] reviewed 21 functional imaging (fMRI and PET) studies involving a pretreatment baseline study and at least one post-treatment follow-up study. Overall, the studies suggested normalization of brain function (i.e., patients were more similar to control subjects following treatment, especially with second-generation antipsychotic drugs), though a wide variability of findings was evident due to methodological limitations such as lack of reliability of data, varying subject populations, research designs, and statistical approaches. Functional imaging can also contribute in pharmacological provocative studies as well as in nonpharmacological behavioral interventions.[100,101]

Conclusions and Recommendations

The field of neuroimaging in psychotic disorders has made progress, especially in schizophrenia, where methods have been initially applied. While there is increased consistency within disorders across methods, there is paucity of work comparing diagnostic specificity of findings. These are exactly the studies required to deconstruct psychosis.

Steps are under way that begin to provide important information: there is a growing literature of structural imaging studies that prospectively examine patients with schizophrenia or bipolar disorder and healthy people, first-episode patients with psychosis followed longitudinally, and family studies of individuals at risk. We have the tools to move the field ahead and need to apply experimental designs that will address fundamental questions. Studies have to include sufficiently large samples to permit clinical correlations and be longitudinal.

Several steps are essential for progress toward the eventual clinical utility of brain imaging in psychiatry. First, collaborating research groups need to standardize their approach to data acquisition, processing, and analyses. This will permit the construction of "atlases" of normal and abnormal brain development. Such "four-dimensional" (3D brains over time) imaging studies must incorporate neurobehavioral paradigms necessary for elucidating brain-behavior relationships most pertinent to these disorders. This approach necessitates multicenter studies in order to obtain sufficiently large samples. Second, we need to incorporate pharmacological probes into fMRI studies because this may provide valuable information linking with molecular substrates and with direct therapeutic implications. Third, cohort studies need to be set up around the time of onset of psychosis to establish the extent to which such abnormalities could be used to define schizophrenia at an early stage, with a view to early intervention and possibly even prevention. These studies could incorporate longitudinal follow-up examinations. Finally, more data are needed to examine the extent to which distinct neuroimaging alterations exist across and within traditional diagnostic boundaries. Such work could inform on whether the observed abnormalities map onto clinical features of symptomatology, course, and treatment response dimensions (the phenome) and to specific genetic polymorphisms (the genome). The availability of such data will permit an evaluation of the usefulness of neuroimaging in the distinction between schizophrenia and affective psychosis and to address a crucial question on how neural activity changes in association with different levels and different types of psychosis.

References

1. Illes J, Kirschen MP, Edwards E, et al. Working group on incidental findings in brain imaging research. Ethics. Incidental findings in brain imaging research. Science. 2006;311:783–784.
2. Lisanby SH, Kohler C, Swanson CL, Gur RE. Psychosis secondary to brain tumor. Semin Clin Neuropsychiatry. 1998;3:1–12.
3. Erhart SM, Young AS, Marder SR, Mintz J. Clinical utility of magnetic resonance imaging radiographs for suspected organic syndromes in adult psychiatry. J Clin Psychiatry. 2005;66:968–973.
4. Lawrie SM, Abukmeil SS, Chiswick A, Egan V, Santosh CG, Best JJ. Qualitative cerebral morphology in schizophrenia: a magnetic resonance imaging study and systematic literature review. Schizophr Res. 1997;25:155–166.

5. Shenton ME, Dickey CC, Frumin M, McCarley RW. A review of MRI findings in schizophrenia. Schizophr Res. 2001;49:1–52.

6. Lawrie SM, Abukmeil SS. Brain abnormality in schizophrenia. A systematic and quantitative review of volumetric magnetic resonance imaging studies. Br J Psychiatry. 1998;172:110–120.

7. Ward KE, Friedman L, Wise A, Schulz SC. Meta-analysis of brain and cranial size in schizophrenia. Schizophr Res. 1996;22:197–213.

8. Wright IC, Rabe-Hesketh S, Woodruff PW, David AS, Murray RM, Bullmore ET. Meta-analysis of regional brain volumes in schizophrenia. Am J Psychiatry. 2000;157:16–25.

9. Woodruff PWR, McManus IC, David AS. Meta-analysis of corpus callosum size in schizophrenia. J Neurol Neurosurg Psychiatry. 1995;58:457–461.

10. Nelson MD, Saykin AJ, Flashman LA, Riordan HJ. Hippocampal volume reduction in schizophrenia as assessed by magnetic resonance imaging: a meta-analytic study. Arch Gen Psychiatry. 1998;55:433–440.

11. Konick LC, Friedman L. Meta-analysis of thalamic size in schizophrenia. Biol Psychiatry. 2001;49:28–38.

12. Davatzikos C, Shen D, Gur RC, et al. Whole brain morphometric study of schizophrenia reveals a spatially complex set of focal abnormalities. Arch Gen Psychiatry. 2005;62:1218–1227.

13. Harrison PJ, Freemantle N, Geddes JR. Meta-analysis of brain weight in schizophrenia. Schizophr Res. 2003;64:25–34.

14. Honea R, Crow TJ, Passingham D, Mackay CE. Regional deficits in brain volume in schizophrenia: a meta-analysis of voxel-based morphometry studies. Am J Psychiatry. 2005;162:2233–2245.

15. Lawrie SM, Johnstone EC, Weinberger DR. Schizophrenia: From Neuroimaging to Neuroscience. Oxford, UK: Oxford University Press; 2004.

16. Antonova E, Sharma T, Morris R, Kumari V. The relationship between brain structure and neurocognition in schizophrenia: a selective review. Schizophr Res. 2004;70:117–145.

17. Scherck H, Falkai P. Effects of antipsychotics on brain structure. Curr Opin Psychiatry. 2006;19:145–150.

18. Vita A, De Peri L, Silenzi C, Dieci M. Brain morphology in first-episode schizophrenia: a meta-analysis of quantitative magnetic resonance imaging studies. Schizophr Res. 2006;82:75–88.

19. Ho BC, Andreasen NC, Nopoulos P, Arndt S, Magnotta V, Flaum M. Progressive structural brain abnormalities and their relationship to clinical outcome: a longitudinal magnetic resonance imaging study early in schizophrenia. Arch Gen Psychiatry. 2003;60:585–594.

20. Hoge EA, Friedman L, Schulz SC. Meta-analysis of brain size in bipolar disorder. Schizophr Res. 1999;37:177–181.

21. Strakowski SM, DelBello MP, Adler C, Cecil DM, Sax KW. Neuroimaging in bipolar disorder. Bipolar Disord. 2000;2:148–164.

22. Bearden CE, Hoffman KM, Cannon TD. The neuropsychology and neuroanatomy of bipolar affective disorder: a critical review. Bipolar Disord. 2001;3:106–150.

23. McDonald C, Zanelli J, Rabe-Hesketh S, et al. Meta-analysis of magnetic resonance imaging brain morphometry studies in bipolar disorder. Biol Psychiatry. 2004;56:411–417.

24. Campbell S, Marriott M, Nahmias C, MacQueen GM. Lower hippocampal volume in patients suffering from depression: a meta-analysis. Am J Psychiatry. 2004;161:598–607.
25. Videbech P, Ravnkilde B. Hippocampal volume and depression: a meta-analysis of MRI studies. Am J Psychiatry. 2004;161:1957–1966.
26. Altshuler LL, Curran JG, Hauser P, Mintz J, Denicoff K, Post R. T2 hyperintensities in bipolar disorder: magnetic resonance imaging comparison and literature meta-analysis. Am J Psychiatry. 1995;152:1139–1144.
27. Videbech P. MRI findings in patients with affective disorder: a meta-analysis. Acta Psychiatr Scand. 1997;96:157–168.
28. Hirayasu Y, Tanaka S, Shenton ME, et al. Prefrontal gray matter volume reduction in first episode schizophrenia. Cereb Cortex. 2001;11:374–381.
29. Dickey CC, Salisbury DF, Nagy AI, et al. Follow-up MRI study of prefrontal volumes in first-episode psychotic patients. Schizophr Res. 2004;71:349–351.
30. Prasad KM, Patel AR, Muddasani S, Sweeney J, Keshavan MS. The entorhinal cortex in first-episode psychotic disorders: a structural magnetic resonance imaging study. Am J Psychiatry. 2004;161:1612–1619.
31. Molina V, Sanz J, Sarramea F, Luque R, Benito C, Palomo T. Dorsolateral prefrontal and superior temporal volume deficits in first-episode psychoses that evolve into schizophrenia. Eur Arch Psychiatry Clin Neurosci. 2006;256:106–111.
32. Wiegand LC, Warfield SK, Levitt JJ, et al. An in vivo MRI study of prefrontal cortical complexity in first-episode psychosis. Am J Psychiatry. 2005;162:65–70.
33. Kanaan RA, Kim JS, Kaufmann WE, Pearlson GD, Barker GJ, McGuire PK. Diffusion tensor imaging in schizophrenia. Biol Psychiatry. 2005;58:921–929.
34. Keshavan MS, Montrose DM, Pierri JN, et al. Magnetic resonance imaging and spectroscopy in offspring at risk for schizophrenia: preliminary studies. Prog Neuropsychopharmacol Biol Psychiatry. 1997;21:1285–1295.
35. Boos HBM, Aleman A, Cahn W, Kahn RS. Brain volumes in relatives of patients with schizophrenia: a meta-analysis. Schizophr Res. 2006;81:41.
36. Job DE, Whalley HC, McConnell S, Glabus MF, Johnstone EC, Lawrie SM. Voxel based morphometry of grey matter densities in subjects at high risk of schizophrenia. Schizophr Res. 2003;64:1–13.
37. Diwadkar VA, Montrose DM, Dworakowski D, Sweeney JA, Keshavan MS. Genetically predisposed offspring with schizotypal features: an ultra high-risk group for schizophrenia? Prog Neuropsychopharmacol Biol Psychiatry. 2006;30:230–238.
38. McIntosh AM, Job DE, Moorhead TW, Harrison LK, Lawrie SM, Johnstone EC. White matter density in patients with schizophrenia, bipolar disorder and their unaffected relatives. Biol Psychiatry. 2005;58:254–257.
39. McDonald C, Bullmore E, Sham P, et al. Regional volume deviations of brain structure in schizophrenia and psychotic bipolar disorder: computational morphometry study. Br J Psychiatry. 2005;186:369–377.
40. McIntosh AM, Job DE, Moorhead WJ, et al. Genetic liability to schizophrenia or bipolar disorder and its relationship to brain structure. Am J Med Genet B Neuropsychiatr Genet. 2006;141:76–83.
41. Phillips LJ, Velakoulis D, Pantelis C, et al. Non-reduction in hippocampal volume is associated with higher risk of psychosis. Schizophr Res. 2002;58:145–158.

42. Pantelis C, Velakoulis D, McGorry PD, et al. Neuroanatomical abnormalities before and after onset of psychosis: a cross-sectional and longitudinal MRI comparison. Lancet. 2003;361:281–288.

43. Job D, Whalley HC, Johnstone EC, Lawrie SM. Grey matter changes over time in high risk subjects developing schizophrenia. Neuroimage. 2005;25:1023–1030.

44. Johnstone EC, Ebmeier KP, Miller P, Owens DGC, Lawrie SM. Predicting schizophrenia—findings from the Edinburgh High Risk Study. Br J Psychiatry. 2005;186:18–25.

45. Velakoulis D, Wood SJ, Wong MT, et al. Hippocampal and amygdala volumes according to psychosis stage and diagnosis: a magnetic resonance imaging study of chronic schizophrenia, first-episode psychosis, and ultra-high-risk individuals. Arch Gen Psychiatry. 2006;63:139–149.

46. Job DE, Whalley HC, McIntosh AM, Johnstone EC, Lawrie SM. Grey matter changes can improve the prediction of schizophrenia in subjects at high risk. BMC Psychiatry. 2006;4:29.

47. Stanley JA, Pettegrew JW, Keshavan MS. Magnetic resonance spectroscopy in schizophrenia: methodological issues and findings–part I. Biol Psychiatry. 2000;48:357–368.

48. Keshavan MS, Stanley JA, Pettegrew JW. Magnetic resonance spectroscopy in schizophrenia: methodological issues and findings–part II. Biol Psychiatry. 2000;48:369–380.

49. Urenjak J, Williams SR, Gadian DG, Noble M. Proton nuclear magnetic resonance spectroscopy unambiguously identifies different neural cell types. J Neurosci. 1993;13:981–989.

50. Rudkin TM, Arnold DL. Proton magnetic resonance spectroscopy for the diagnosis and management of cerebral disorders. Arch Neurol. 1999;56:919–926.

51. Baslow MH. Functions of N-acetyl-L-aspartate and N-acetyl-L-aspartylglutamate in the vertebrate brain: role in glial cell-specific signaling. J Neurochem. 2000;75:453–459.

52. Lim KO, Adalsteinsson E, Spielman D, Sullivan EV, Rosenbloom MJ, Pfefferbaum A. Proton magnetic resonance spectroscopic imaging of cortical gray and white matter in schizophrenia. Arch Gen Psychiatry. 1998;55:346–352.

53. Tsai G, Coyle JT. N-acetylaspartate in neuropsychiatric disorders. Prog Neurobiol. 1995;46:531–540.

54. Steen RG, Hamer RM, Lieberman JA. Measurement of brain metabolites by 1H magnetic resonance spectroscopy in patients with schizophrenia: a systematic review and meta-analysis. Neuropsychopharmacology. 2005;30:1949–1962.

55. Ende G, Braus DF, Walter S, et al. Effects of age, medication, and illness duration on the N-acetyl aspartate signal of the anterior cingulate region in schizophrenia. Schizophr Res. 2000;41:389–395.

56. Yildiz-Yesiloglu A, Ankerst DP. Neurochemical alterations of the brain in bipolar disorder and their implications for pathophysiology: a systematic review of the in vivo proton magnetic resonance spectroscopy findings. Prog Neuropsychopharmacol Biol Psychiatry. 2006;30:969–995.

57. Yildiz-Yesiloglu A, Ankerst DP. Review of 1H magnetic resonance spectroscopy findings in major depressive disorder: a meta-analysis. Psychiatry Res. 2006;147:1–25.

58. Callicott JH, Egan MF, Bertolino A, et al. Hippocampal N-acetyl aspartate in unaffected siblings of patients with schizophrenia: a possible intermediate neurobiological phenotype. Biol Psychiatry. 1998;44:941–950.
59. Tibbo P, Hanstock C, Valiakalayil A, Allen P. 3-T proton MRS investigation of glutamate and glutamine in adolescents at high genetic risk for schizophrenia. Am J Psychiatry. 2004;161:1116–1118.
60. Jessen F, Scherk H, Traber F, et al. Proton magnetic resonance spectroscopy in subjects at risk for schizophrenia. Schizophr Res. 2006;87:81–88.
61. Wood SJ, Berger G, Velakoulis D, et al. Proton magnetic resonance spectroscopy in first episode psychosis and ultra high-risk individuals. Schizophr Bull. 2003;29:831–843.
62. Pettegrew JW, Keshavan MS, Panchalingam K, et al. Alterations in brain high-energy phosphate and membrane phospholipid metabolism in first-episode, drug-naive schizophrenics. A pilot study of the dorsal prefrontal cortex by in vivo phosphorus 31 nuclear magnetic resonance spectroscopy. Arch Gen Psychiatry. 1991;48:563–568.
63. Stanley JA, Williamson PC, Drost DJ, et al. An in vivo study of the prefrontal cortex of schizophrenic patients at different stages of illness via phosphorus magnetic resonance spectroscopy. Arch Gen Psychiatry. 1995;52:399–406.
64. Fukuzako H, Fukuzako T, Hashiguchi T, Kodama S, Takigawa M, Fujimoto T. Changes in levels of phosphorus metabolites in temporal lobes of drug-naive schizophrenic patients. Am J Psychiatry. 1999;156:1205–1208.
65. Jensen JE, Miller J, Williamson PC, et al. Focal changes in brain energy and phospholipid metabolism in first-episode schizophrenia: ^{31}P-MRS chemical shift imaging study at 4 Tesla. Br J Psychiatry. 2004;184:409–415.
66. Berger GE, Wood SJ, Pantelis C, Velakoulis D, Wellard RM, McGorry PD. Implications of lipid biology for the pathogenesis of schizophrenia. Aust NZ J Psychiatry. 2002;36:355–366.
67. Klemm S, Rzanny R, Riehemann S, et al. Cerebral phosphate metabolism in first-degree relatives of patients with schizophrenia. Am J Psychiatry. 2001;158:958–960.
68. Keshavan MS, Haas G, Miewald J, et al. Prolonged untreated illness duration from prodromal onset predicts outcome in first episode psychoses. Schizophr Bull. 2003;29:757–769.
69. Kato T, Takahashi S, Shioiri T, Inubushi T. Alterations in brain phosphorous metabolism in bipolar disorder detected by in vivo 31P and 7Li magnetic resonance spectroscopy. J Affect Disord. 1993;27:53–59.
70. Wong DF, Wagner HN Jr, Tune LE, et al. Positron emission tomography reveals elevated D2 dopamine receptors in drug-naive schizophrenics. Science. 1986;234:1558–1563.
71. Farde L, Wiesel FA, Hall H, Halldin C, Stone-Elander S, Sedvall G. No D2 receptor increase in PET study of schizophrenia. Arch Gen Psychiatry. 1987;44:671–672.
72. Andreasen NC, Carson R, Diksic M, et al. Workshop on schizophrenia, PET, and dopamine D2 receptors in the human neostriatum. Schizophr Bull. 1988;14:471–484.
73. Zakzanis KK, Hansen KT. Dopamine D2 densities and the schizophrenic brain. Schizophr Res. 1998;32:201–206.
74. Laruelle M. Imaging dopamine transmission in schizophrenia. A review and meta-analysis. Q J Nucl Med. 1998;42:211–221.

75. Erritzoe D, Talbot P, Frankle WG, Abi-Dargham A. Positron emission tomography and single photon emission CT molecular imaging in schizophrenia. Neuroimaging Clin N Am. 2003;13:817–832.

76. Abi-Dargham A. Do we still believe in the dopamine hypothesis? New data bring new evidence. Int J Neuropsychopharmacol. 2004;7(Suppl 1):S1–S5.

77. Cropley VL, Fujita M, Innis RB, Nathan PJ. Molecular imaging of the dopaminergic system and its association with human cognitive function. Biol Psychiatry. 2006;59:898–907.

78. Cannon DM, Ichise M, Fromm SJ, et al. Serotonin transporter binding in bipolar disorder assessed using [11C]DASB and positron emission tomography. Biol Psychiatry. 2006;60:207–217.

79. Cannon DM, Carson RE, Nugent AC, et al. Reduced muscarinic type 2 receptor binding in subjects with bipolar disorder. Arch Gen Psychiatry. 2006;63:741–747.

80. Talbott PS, Laruelle M. The role of in vivo molecular imaging with PET and SPECT in the elucidation of psychiatric drug action and new drug development. Eur Neuropsychopharmacol. 2002;12:503–511.

81. Tauscher J, Kapur S. Choosing the right dose of antipsychotics in schizophrenia: lessons from neuroimaging studies. CNS Drugs. 2001;15:671–678.

82. Gur RE, Gur RC. Neuroimaging in schizophrenia: linking neuropsychiatric manifestations to neurobiology. In: Kaplan HI, Sadock BJ, eds. Comprehensive Textbook of Psychiatry/VIII. Philadelphia, PA: Lippincott Williams and Wilkins; 2005:1396–1407.

83. Zakzanis KK, Heinrichs RW. Schizophrenia and the frontal brain: a quantitative review. J Int Neuropsychol Soc. 1999;5:556–566.

84. Hill K, Mann L, Laws KR, Stephenson CM, Nimmo-Smith I, McKenna PJ. Hypofrontality in schizophrenia: a meta-analysis of functional imaging studies. Acta Psychiatr Scand. 2004;110:243–256.

85. Davidson LL, Heinrichs RW. Quantification of frontal and temporal lobe brain-imaging findings in schizophrenia: a meta-analysis. Psychiatry Res. 2003;122:69–87.

86. Achim AM, Lepage M. Episodic memory-related activation in schizophrenia: meta-analysis. Br J Psychiatry. 2005;187:500–509.

87. Glahn DC, Ragland JD, Abramoff A, et al. Beyond hypofrontality: a quantitative meta-analysis of functional neuroimaging studies of working memory in schizophrenia. Hum Brain Mapp. 2005;25:60–69.

88. Davis CE, Jeste DV, Eyler LT. Review of longitudinal functional neuroimaging studies of drug treatments in patients with schizophrenia. Schizophr Res. 2005;78:45–60.

89. MacDonald AW 3rd, Carter CS, Kerns JG, et al. Specificity of prefrontal dysfunction and context processing deficits to schizophrenia in never-medicated patients with first-episode psychosis. Am J Psychiatry. 2005;162:475–484.

90. Zakzanis KK, Poulin P, Hansen KT, Jolic D. Searching the schizophrenic brain for temporal lobe deficits: a systematic review and meta-analysis. Psychol Med. 2000;30:491–504.

91. Friston KJ, Frith CD. Schizophrenia: a disconnection syndrome? Clin Neurosci. 1995;3:89–97.

92. Stephan KE, Baldeweg T, Friston KJ. Synaptic plasticity and dysconnection in schizophrenia. Biol Psychiatry. 2006;59:929–939.

93. Uhlhaas PJ, Linden DE, Singer W, et al. Dysfunctional long-range coordination of neural activity during Gestalt perception in schizophrenia. J Neurosci. 2006;26:8168–8175.

94. Uhlhaas PJ, Singer W. Neural synchrony in brain disorders: relevance for cognitive dysfunctions and pathophysiology. Neuron. 2006;52:155–168.

95. Whalley HC, Whyte MC, Johnstone EC, Lawrie SM. Neural correlates of enhanced genetic risk for schizophrenia. Neuroscientist. 2005;11:238–249.

96. Spence SA, Liddle PF, Stefan MD, et al. Functional anatomy of verbal fluency in people with schizophrenia and those at genetic risk. Focal dysfunction and distributed disconnectivity reappraised. Br J Psychiatry. 2000;176:52–60.

97. Whalley HC, Simonotto E, Marshall I, et al. Functional disconnectivity in subjects at high genetic risk of schizophrenia. Brain. 2005;128:2097–2108.

98. Whalley HC, Simonotto E, Moorhead W, et al. Functional imaging as a predictor of schizophrenia. Biol Psychiatry. 2006;60:454–462.

99. Wolf DH, Gur RC, Valdez JN, et al. Alterations of frontotemporal connectivity during word encoding in schizophrenia. Psychiatry Res. 2007;154:221–232.

100. Wexler BE, Anderson M, Fulbright RK, Gore JC. Preliminary evidence of improved verbal working memory performance and normalization of task-related frontal lobe activation in schizophrenia following cognitive exercises. Am J Psychiatry. 2000;157:1694–1697.

101. Wykes T, Brammer M, Mellers J, et al. Effects on the brain of a psychological treatment: cognitive remediation therapy: functional magnetic resonance imaging in schizophrenia. Br J Psychiatry. 2002;181:144–152.

10

IDENTIFYING FUNCTIONAL NEUROIMAGING BIOMARKERS OF BIPOLAR DISORDER

Toward DSM-V

Mary L. Phillips, M.D., MRCPsych
Eduard Vieta, M.D., Ph.D.

Bipolar disorder remains one of the 10 most debilitating illnesses worldwide,[1] with a prevalence of at least 1%. Bipolar-1 disorder (BP-1), characterized by the presence of episodes of mania and depression, in particular is associated with a poor clinical and functional outcome, a high suicide rate,[2] and a huge societal cost.[3] One reason for the poor prognosis is the frequent misdiagnosis or late diagnosis of the disorder,[4,5] leading to delays in the initiation of appropriate treatment. Indeed, while depression is a more common presentation and a cause of greater disruption of occupational, family, and social functioning than mania in individuals with bipolar disorder,[6] bipolar depression continues to be frequently misdiag-

Reprinted with permission from Phillips ML, Vieta E. "Identifying Functional Neuroimaging Biomarkers of Bipolar Disorder: Toward DSM-V." *Schizophrenia Bulletin* 2007; 33: 893–904.

nosed and inappropriately treated as unipolar depression in individuals without a clear previous history of manic episodes.[7–10] Increased accuracy in diagnosing bipolar disorder in individuals when they present during depression therefore remains a key goal to help improve the mental health, treatment, and clinical and functional outcomes of individuals with all subtypes of the disorder.

The recent research agenda for *Diagnostic and Statistical Manual of Mental Disorders,* 5th Edition (DSM-V), has emphasized a need to translate basic and clinical neuroscience research findings into a new classification system for all psychiatric disorders based upon pathophysiological and etiological processes.[11–14] These pathophysiological processes involve complex relationships between genetic variables, abnormalities in brain systems, and related neuropsychological function and behavior and may be represented as biomarkers of a disorder.[15] Abnormalities that are persistent rather than episodic or state features of a disorder can be more readily used to identify those individuals with the disorder.[16] Measurement in individuals with bipolar disorder of brain system abnormalities underlying characteristic behavioral impairments that are "common to remission and depression" may therefore help to identify future biomarkers of the disorder,[17,18] as will examination of brain system abnormalities that are "specific to bipolar disorder" and not common to unipolar depression. These studies will facilitate future increases in accuracy of diagnosis of bipolar disorder and subsequent treatment improvements in depressed individuals presenting without a clear history of mania.

There may be several different symptom domains in the traditional BP-1.[14] One important symptom domain is mood instability leading to variability in depression and/or hypomanic/manic states as well as other aspects of mood variability that might be expressed as irritability or sadness. This may be related to impaired processing of emotionally salient information in the environment. A second major symptom domain is impaired cognitive control and executive dysfunction, which includes symptoms such as the inability to concentrate, difficulty in decision making, and memory difficulties. Together, these two symptom domains may confer an inability to regulate emotional states in any given context, as individuals are unable to employ appropriate cognitive control processes, including reappraisal, suppression, or inhibitory processes,[19] either with or without overt awareness, to regulate and inhibit the generation of inappropriate emotional states. Subsyndromal levels of these symptom domains persist during remission in individuals with the disorder[20] and may underlie the vulnerability to subsequent severe mood episodes.[21] Thus, examination of activity in neural systems associated with 1) initial identification and generation of emotional states in response to emotionally salient material and 2) covert and overt cognitive control processes that may be linked with the ability to regulate emotional states[22] is a first stage toward the longer term goal of identifying biomarkers of bipolar disorder.

We therefore next describe experimental paradigms that can be employed in neuroimaging studies to measure activity in neural systems associated with these two major symptom domains in bipolar disorder. These include neural systems underlying 1) emotion processing, specifically, neural systems implicated in the initial identification and generation of emotional states in response to emotionally salient material and 2) cognitive control processes, including attention, working memory, inhibitory control, strategy development, and cognitive flexibility.[23] Abnormal function in these two neural systems may be linked, respectively, with the mood instability and impaired cognitive control processes that are commonly observed in bipolar disorder. We therefore subsequently describe the functional abnormalities in these neural systems that have been reported in bipolar disorder using paradigms designed specifically to examine activity in these neural systems and the extent to which these abnormalities may be specific to bipolar disorder rather than being common to unipolar depression.

Paradigms Measuring Neural Responses During Emotion Processing, Working Memory, Attention, and Emotion Regulation

Paradigms to examine activity associated with the first symptom domain, mood instability, that may be associated with impaired processing of emotionally salient information have included displays of facial expressions. These stimuli are highly salient social signals of emotional states, the correct recognition of which is crucial for social interaction. Facial expression identification tasks have therefore been widely used in the examination of emotion-processing abilities in healthy and psychiatric populations.[21,24] In healthy individuals, findings from neuroimaging studies have implicated a network of subcortical, predominantly anterior limbic regions in response to presentations of different facial expressions, including ventral striatum, amygdala, anterior hippocampus, and anterior insula.[24–28] Numerous other types of emotional stimuli have been employed in the examination of neural systems implicated in emotion processing. These include emotional scenes, emotional words, and emotional material presented in different sensory modalities.[21]

The second symptom domain, impaired cognitive control and executive dysfunction, maps to dysfunction in a lateral prefrontal cortical system, comprising dorsolateral and ventrolateral prefrontal cortex (DLPFC and VLPFC), which is important for cognitive and executive function (e.g., Monchi et al.[29]), and the hippocampus, important for memory. One commonly employed task of working memory and attention is the digit-sorting task. This task requires the sorting of digits into numerical order and memorization of the digit with the middle value. The performance of this task has been reliably associated with DLPFC activity in healthy individuals.[30] Numerous studies employing attentional tasks, including the Stroop interference task, in which individuals selectively attend to the color ink in which a color word is written rather than the color word per se, have further implicated the DLPFC,[31] dorsal regions of the anterior cingulate gyrus,[32–35] and ventral prefrontal cortex (VPFC)[36] during performance of these tasks in healthy individuals.

Fewer studies have specifically focused on examination of neural systems underlying regulation of emotion. Recent studies have implicated dorsal prefrontal cortical regions both in the suppression of arousal to emotive stimuli[37] and reappraisal of emotive scenes[19,39] during attempts to reduce emotional experience. Another method of examining emotion regulatory processes less confounded by interindividual differences in emotion regulatory strategies is to employ paradigms measuring the impact of emotional contexts upon subsequent performance of executive control or attentional tasks. This method has previously been employed in healthy individuals and those with unipolar depression,[30] with findings indicating reciprocal relationships between amygdala and dorsolateral prefrontal cortical responses during the attentional component of such tasks. Clearly, further study is required in healthy individuals of the nature of neural systems that are specifically implicated in the different cognitive control processes implicated in emotional state regulation.

In the following sections, evidence is presented for abnormalities in neural response during performance of these tasks in remitted individuals with bipolar disorder compared with healthy individuals. Findings are then described from studies examining neural responses during these tasks in depressed individuals with bipolar disorder compared with healthy individuals, and in depressed individuals compared with remitted individuals with bipolar disorder, to examine the extent to which such abnormalities are common in remission and depression.

Functional Abnormalities in Neural Systems Underlying Emotion Processing and Cognitive Control Processes in Bipolar Remission

The few existing studies examining neural responses to emotional stimuli have indicated increased amygdala and ventral striatal activity to mild happy[39] and intense fearful expressions[39,40] in remitted, and increased amygdala activity to happy expressions in a mixed group of remitted and unwell,[41] individuals with bipolar disorder. Findings also show decreased DLPFC activity to fearful expressions[38] in remitted individuals with bipolar disorder (predominantly the bipolar I subtype) compared with healthy individuals. No significant relationship between subsyndromal depression severity and amygdala responses to happy and fearful facial expressions has been observed in remitted individuals with bipolar disorder.[39] Interestingly, other studies have demonstrated widespread decreases in prefrontal cortical and subcortical neural activity to emotional words in remitted individuals with BP-1.[42,43] It is therefore possible that emotional facial expressions are processed as particularly significant in individuals with bipolar disorders during remission.

During performance of attentional tasks, findings in remitted, euthymic individuals with bipolar disorder compared with healthy individuals have indicated reduced activity in dorsal and ventral prefrontal cortical regions[36] and reduced activity within dorsal regions of the anterior cingulate gyrus, although increased DLPFC activity,[44] during a Stroop interference task. Other studies have demonstrated reduced DLPFC activity in euthymic individuals with bipolar disorder during working memory and verbal encoding tasks.[45,46] Increases in activity within subcortical regions associated with emotion processing rather than working memory or attention have also been demonstrated in remitted, euthymic individuals with bipolar disorder during performance of a continuous performance task[47] and a working memory task[48] and in adolescents with bipolar disorder during performance of a Stroop attentional task.[49]

These findings suggest "increased amygdala and subcortical" activity but predominantly "decreased DLPFC" activity during emotion-processing and cognitive control tasks in bipolar remission. There are some inconsistencies that may relate to the nature of the emotional stimuli employed in these tasks. Findings indicate that facial expressions may be processed as particularly salient stimuli in remitted individuals with bipolar disorder. We next describe findings from studies examining neural responses during these tasks in bipolar depression.

Are There Functional Abnormalities in Neural Systems Common to Bipolar Remission and Depression?

Findings indicate increased subcortical activity to negative scenes during the generation of emotional states in bipolar depressed individuals (including rapid cycling) compared with healthy individuals,[50] and decreased activity in medial prefrontal cortex during sad mood induction in remitted[51] more than depressed bipolar individuals.[52] One study has reported relative increases in activity in a number of subcortical regions to happy facial expressions in bipolar depressed compared with manic individuals and healthy individuals,[53] but further study focused upon amygdala and prefrontal cortical responses is required in larger numbers of bipolar depressed and remitted individuals. Increased amygdala activity has been demonstrated in both bipolar depressed and remitted individuals (approximately 50% type I) compared with healthy individuals at rest.[54] During a sustained attention task, findings have indicated decreased absolute prefrontal cortical and increased subcortical metabolism, with negative and positive correlations between metabolism in these prefrontal cortical and subcortical regions, respectively, and depression severity in bipolar depressed (predominantly rapid cycling) compared with healthy individuals.[55]

Of the few studies directly comparing neural activity during performance of attentional tasks in remitted or euthymic versus depressed individuals with bipolar disorder, relative increases in ventrolateral prefrontal cortical activity have been reported in bipolar depressed compared with euthymic individuals during performance of a Stroop task.[36] Similarly, during performance of a Stroop attentional task, depression severity correlated negatively with the magnitude of the ventral prefrontal cortical decreases in individuals with bipolar disorder.[56] These findings suggest common functional abnormalities in subcortical and prefrontal cortical regions during bipolar depression and remission compared with healthy individuals. They also indicate further depression-related abnormalities, in particular, relative increases in prefrontal cortical activity during attentional tasks in bipolar depressed compared with remitted individuals. Further study is required to identify abnormal neural responses during emotion-processing, attentional, and working memory tasks and tasks involving emotion regulatory processes, which persist and are therefore common to remission and depression in bipolar disorder. Current data comparing bipolar depressed and remitted individuals suggest a positive association between increased prefrontal cortical activity and increased depression severity during attentional tasks.

There is a lack of studies specifically examining the relationship between change in depression severity over time in individuals with bipolar disorder and change in the nature and magnitude of abnormal neural activity during emotion and cognitive challenge tasks. This seriously limits current understanding of the neural mechanisms associated with change in depression severity over time in bipolar depression. Longitudinal examination of the relationship between depression severity and abnormal neural activity is therefore required to better understand these neural mechanisms. Another problem is the paucity of studies comparing neural activity during emotion and cognitive challenge tasks in bipolar and unipolar depressed populations. This limits understanding of the extent to which abnormalities observed in bipolar depression are bipolar specific or depression related and therefore common to both bipolar and unipolar populations. We next describe findings from studies that have employed these tasks in unipolar depressed compared with healthy individuals and the few findings from studies that have directly compared neural activity in bipolar and unipolar populations.

The Link With Mania:
Are There Similar Functional Neural Abnormalities Evident in Mania, Depression, and Remission in Bipolar Disorder?

A clear history of mania indicates a diagnosis of bipolar disorder rather than unipolar depression. To fully understand the pathophysiological mechanisms underlying bipolar disorder, it is important to consider the nature of functional abnormalities in neural systems that may persist across mania, depression, and remission. Few studies have examined activity in neural systems associated with the two symptom domains in individuals during mania. To date, studies have reported in manic individuals relative to healthy individuals increased amygdala,[57] insula,[58] and subcortical activity per se[53] in response to negative emotional facial expressions and to negative scenes,[59] increased ventral striatal activity at rest[60] and during motor tasks,[61] and decreased ventral prefrontal cortical activity during performance of a variety of different cognitive control tasks.[62–65] Together with findings from functional neuroimaging studies of depressed and remitted individuals with bipolar disorder, these data suggest patterns of increased amygdala and subcortical activity in response to emotional—at least negative emotional—stimuli and decreases in activity in prefrontal cortical regions implicated in cognitive control processes that may be common to all three phases of bipolar illness. More study is required, however, examining the nature of functional abnormalities in emotion-processing neural systems to different categories of emotional stimuli (e.g., positive vs. negative emotional stimuli) and during different cognitive control tasks in individuals during mania.

Abnormal Neural Responses in Unipolar Depressed Individuals

The majority of functional neuroimaging studies of unipolar depressed individuals pre- and postremission after treatment with pharmacological and psychological interventions have been performed during resting state and not during performance of specific emotion-processing or attentional tasks.[66–75] There are discrepant findings from these studies. Some studies report increases in dorsal and ventral prefrontal cortical activity[66,67,71,75,76] or decreases in subcortical and ventral prefrontal cortical responses[73] in unipolar depressed individuals and in mixed groups of individuals with unipolar and bipolar depression after depression improvement with pharmacological intervention. Other studies suggest decreases in dorsolateral and ventrolateral prefrontal cortical activity after successful psychological and pharmacological interventions[68,70,74,77] or relative increases only in subcortical, limbic regions after both types of intervention in unipolar depressed individuals.[73] Studies have also reported an inverse relationship between depression severity and dorsal prefrontal cortical and anterior cingulate gyral activity in unipolar depressed individuals at rest.[66,78] Regarding neural responses during performance of emotion-processing tasks, abnormal increases in amygdala or ventral striatal activity have been demonstrated by unipolar depressed individuals in response to negative emotional expressions,[79–81] and similar patterns of decreased ventromedial prefrontal activity during sad mood induction compared with healthy individuals have been reported in unipolar remitted and depressed individuals.[82] Decreased activity in left DLPFC relative to healthy individuals has been reported in unipolar depressed individuals during working memory trials following negative stimuli[30] and during working memory and attention.[83–85] In the majority of studies, an amelioration of the abnormal pattern of neural response during depression has been demonstrated in unipolar depressed individuals after remission. For example, abnormal increases in amygdala or ventral striatal activity in response to negative emotional expressions in unipolar depressed individuals[79–81] significantly reduce in remission after treatment with antidepressant medication.[79,80] Increases after remission in insular and anterior cingulate gyral activity in response to negative versus neutral scenes have also been reported.[86]

In summary, while findings regarding neural responses during at-rest studies are somewhat discrepant in unipolar depressed individuals, findings from studies employing emotional challenge paradigms suggest that, similar to individuals with bipolar disorder, unipolar depressed individuals show increased amygdala and sub-cortical activity in response to emotional stimuli relative to healthy individuals. Unlike individuals with bipolar disorder, however, in unipolar depressed individuals this abnormal pattern of neural activity is predominantly negative rather than positive emotional stimuli. Furthermore, these abnormalities appear to be *depression dependent* in unipolar depressed individuals rather than abnormalities common throughout depression and remission. Only one study to date has directly compared neural activity in bipolar and unipolar individuals. Here, we showed increases in amygdala and subcortical activity in response not only to mild happy expressions but also to fearful facial expressions versus neutral expressions in remitted bipolar relative to unipolar depressed individuals.[39] There is thus clearly a need for studies comparing neural activity in bipolar and unipolar populations during emotional and cognitive challenge paradigms, but data to date suggest that examination of patterns of subcortical neural activity in response to negative and positive stimuli may help distinguish individuals with bipolar disorder from those with unipolar depression. Furthermore, there is a need to examine the extent to which relationships between changes in depression severity over time and changes in neural activity differentiate bipolar and unipolar populations.

A Neural Model of Bipolar Disorder

Current findings require replication in larger numbers of participants but suggest that bipolar disorder can be modeled as dysfunction in two neural systems that are implicated in two major symptom domains in bipolar disorder: 1) abnormally increased activity in an amygdala- and subcortical-centered system underlying emotion processing that may be linked with the mood instability commonly observed in individuals with bipolar disorder and 2) abnormally decreased activity in a pre-

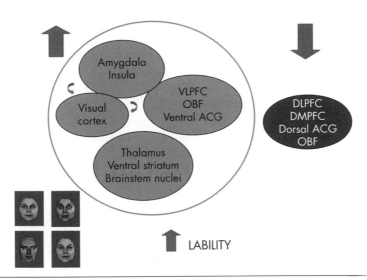

FIGURE 10–1. Schematic model for the neural basis of the affective instability in individuals with bipolar disorder.

In bipolar disorder, it is postulated that, in response to many emotional stimuli including the different categories of facial expression depicted here, although not consistently to emotional words, a pattern of increased activity occurs in an amygdala- and subcortical-centered neural system important for the identification of emotional information and the generation of emotional states *(depicted in dark gray)*. This, together with reduced activity in a DLPFC- and VLPFC-centered system important for cognitive control processes involved in the regulation of behavioral responses to emotional stimuli *(depicted in light gray)*, may lead to impaired emotion regulation and increased lability of mood frequently observed in individuals with bipolar disorder.

ACG=anterior cingulate gyrus; DLPFC=dorsolateral prefrontal cortex; DMPFC=dorsomedial prefrontal cortex; OBF=orbitofrontal cortex; VLPFC=ventrolateral prefrontal cortex.

frontal cortical neural system comprising predominantly DLPFC and VPFC underlying cognitive control processes, including attention, working memory, inhibitory control, strategy development, and cognitive flexibility,[21,23,29] that may be linked with impaired cognitive control and executive dysfunction observed in bipolar disorder (Figure 10–1). The former (1) may underlie the emotional lability, the latter (2) the impaired attention and distractibility, and the combination of both abnormalities, the inability to employ cognitive control strategies, either with covert or overt awareness, to successfully regulate emotional states that are common clinical features of bipolar disorder. While functional regulation of the amygdala may be directly mediated by ventromedial prefrontal cortex,[87] functional abnormalities in these two neural systems are suggested by the few functional neuroimaging studies to date in bipolar disorder. Findings suggest that abnormalities described in (1) to emotional stimuli may occur both in remitted[39] and depressed[53] bipolar individuals, but no studies have directly compared neural activity during emotion-processing paradigms in these two populations. Findings further suggest relative increases in activity in the prefrontal cortical-centered system in bipolar depression compared with bipolar remission during attention tasks.[36,54] In unipolar depression, unlike bipolar disorder, findings suggest that abnormalities described in (1) above may occur in response to some negative, but not positive, emotional stimuli and may thus distinguish bipolar from unipolar populations[39,69] (Table 10–1). To date, only one study has directly compared bipolar and unipolar individuals[39] and provides some support for this potential distinction between bipolar remitted and unipolar depressed individuals. Clearly, there is a need for far more research in this burgeoning area of clinical neuroscience. Specifically, future studies should focus on the employment of experimental paradigms to examine the nature of functional abnormalities in the two neural systems described above that map closely to common symptom domains in bipolar disorder and the extent to which these abnormalities may help distinguish individuals with bipolar disorder, especially when presenting during depressed episode, from individuals with unipolar depression.

The Effect of Structural Volume Abnormalities, Medication, and Other Clinical Variables Upon Functional Neural Abnormalities

Here, we describe other factors that may have an impact upon measurements of functional neural response during task performance in individuals with bipolar disorder (some findings including other bipolar subtypes), but which remain relatively unexamined. These include effects of regional structural neural volume abnormalities, psychotropic medication, and other clinical variables, including illness duration, subsyndromal symptoms of depression and mania in remitted individuals with bipolar disorder, comorbid anxiety, history of psychotic symptoms, and history of alcohol and illicit substance abuse. Regarding regional structural volume abnormalities, findings have indicated amygdala volume increases in adult individuals with bipolar disorder[90–93] but decreases in adolescent individuals with BP-1.[94–100] Other studies have reported increased ventral striatal (caudate nucleus and putamen) volumes[92,98,100] and decreased anterior thalamic volumes.[101] In contrast, smaller amygdala (and hippocampal) volumes have been more consistently reported in unipolar depressed individuals.[102–104] Findings regarding prefrontal cortical volumes have indicated decreased volume and gray matter density in anterior cingulate and subgenual cingulate gyri[105–108] and dorsal prefrontal cortex and VPFC[91,107,109–111] and reduced density in the right subgenual anterior cin-

TABLE 10–1. Neural activity during emotion and cognitive challenge tasks in bipolar disorder and unipolar depression

	Bipolar remitted	Bipolar depressed	Bipolar mania	Unipolar depressed
Emotion processing	Increased amygdala and ventral striatal activity in response to positive and negative stimuli	Increased amygdala and ventral striatal activity in response to positive and negative stimuli	Increased amygdala and ventral striatal activity in response to negative emotional stimuli	Increased amygdala activity in response to negative, but not positive, stimuli
Cognitive control tasks	Decreased subcortical activity in response to emotional words	Increased DLPFC and VPFC activity relative to bipolar remitted	Decreased VPFC activity	Decreased DLPFC and VPFC activity

Note. DLPFC=dorsolateral prefrontal cortex; VPFC=ventral prefrontal cortex.

gulate and adjacent white matter in individuals with bipolar disorder compared with healthy individuals.[112] Recent findings further indicate gray matter volume reductions in the lateral orbitofrontal cortex of medicated individuals with bipolar subtypes I and II compared with healthy individuals.[113] There have also been reports of no significant differences in prefrontal cortical volumes between individuals with bipolar disorder and healthy individuals, however.[114,115] Similar patterns of reduced prefrontal cortical volume have been shown in unipolar depressed individuals,[102,116–118] particularly elderly unipolar depressed individuals.[119] Overall, while findings indicate structural volume abnormalities in amygdala and prefrontal cortical volumes,[120] a recent meta-analysis has indicated that the most consistent structural abnormality is an increase in right ventricular volume in individuals with bipolar disorder.[121]

Mood-stabilizing medications, including divalproex sodium and lithium, have been reported as either decreasing prefrontal cortical blood flow or having no effect. In healthy individuals, benzodiazepine dose inversely correlates with amygdala response to facial expressions,[122] while acute administration of selective serotonin reuptake inhibitor antidepressant medication has been associated with decreased amygdalar response to fearful facial expressions and aversive scenes[123–125] and a suppressed electrophysiological response in frontal and occipital cortices to unpleasant scenes.[126] Administration of the atypical neuroleptic sultopride has been associated with decreased amygdalar response to aversive compared with neutral scenes in healthy individuals.[124] In bipolar depressed individuals, antidepressant medication has been associated with relative increases in prefrontal cortical metabolism at rest.[66] Mood stabilizer medication has been associated with relative decreases in amygdala activity in remitted individuals with bipolar disorder (50% type I) at rest[54] and decreases in amygdala activity in a mixed group of remitted and unwell individuals with bipolar disorder to emotional facial expressions.[41] Other studies have shown a significant positive correlation between neuroleptic medication dose (in chlorpromazine equivalents) and activity in rostral anterior cingulate gyrus and DLPFC in remitted, euthymic individuals with BP-1[44] and increased DLPFC activity in medicated compared with unmedicated euthymic individuals with bipolar disorder [127] during Stroop task performance, although no significant effect of any psychotropic medication was reported in individuals with bipolar disorder during a working memory task.[48] Long-term psychotropic medication use[113] and antidepressant exposure[109] have been associated with relative decreases in ventral prefrontal cortical gray matter volume in individuals with bipolar disorder, but long-term effects of psychotropic medication upon regional structural volumes remain unclear.[128,129] The effect of medication upon neural responses during task performance in bipolar populations therefore requires further study.

Together, these findings indicate structural abnormalities in prefrontal cortical and subcortical regions that are components of neural systems implicated in two symptom domains of bipolar disorder. Furthermore, psychotropic medications that are commonly taken by individuals with bipolar disorder may impact activity, at least in part, in these neural regions of interest in individuals with bipolar disorder. As there is so little study of the nature of structural-functional relationships in these neural regions or the effect of psychotropic medication upon activity in these regions in bipolar study, these remain important areas for future research.

Future Research: Can We Identify Biomarkers of Risk for Bipolar Disorder?

Elucidation of neural system abnormalities that are persistent and bipolar disorder specific remains a main focus of research aiming to identify biomarkers of bipolar disorder. A subsequent stage will be the examination of the extent to which these abnormalities are shared with bipolar subtypes other than the traditional bipolar I subtype.[129,130] Another goal for longer term, future research in bipolar disorder that reflects major clinical problems associated with the disorder is the identification of biomarkers that allow us to predict the degree of risk of subsequent development of bipolar disorder in individuals who are at risk for, but as yet undiagnosed with, the disorder.

Findings from studies examining neural system abnormalities in bipolar disorder will ultimately lead to future studies examining the extent to which such neural system abnormalities exist as potential biomarkers of risk for bipolar disorder. Thus, future research should focus on examination of neural system abnormalities that are common to individuals with bipolar disorder and those as yet undiagnosed with the disorder (e.g., individuals presenting with depression but yet to develop a manic or hypomanic episode), and individuals at high genetic risk for the disorder (e.g., offspring and as yet unaffected siblings of individuals with bipolar disorder). Only one study to date has examined functional neural abnormalities in individuals with bipolar disorder and their healthy siblings.[51] In this study, the authors measured regional cerebral blood flow (rCBF) with [^{15}O] water positron emission tomography after induction of transient sadness in nine euthymic individuals with bipolar disorder who had responded to lithium and nine healthy siblings. Common to both groups and a group of individuals with bipolar disorder who had responded to sodium valproate were rCBF increases in the dorsal/rostral anterior cingulate and anterior insula and decreases in the orbitofrontal and inferior temporal cortices. The authors noted that changes in rCBF during sadness induction were not seen previously in healthy subjects without a family history of mood disorder. The study's findings are therefore a first stage toward the identification of biomarkers of risk for bipolar disorder. Another study has demonstrated an association between genetic risk for bipolar disorder (in healthy siblings of adults with bipolar disorder) with gray matter volume deficits specifically within the right anterior cingulate gyrus and ventral striatum.[131]

To date, there have been no studies examining neural system abnormalities in healthy offspring of individuals with bipolar disorder. One study has, however, examined neurochemical abnormalities in offspring diagnosed with mood disorders (but not bipolar disorder) of adults with bipolar disorder using proton magnetic resonance spectroscopy.[132] Similar to findings in adults with bipolar disorders, neurochemical abnormalities were demonstrated within frontal cortex and cerebellar vermis in these offspring. There is clearly much scope for future research to employ different functional neuroimaging techniques to examine potential biomarkers of risk for bipolar disorder.

Conclusion

The recent research agenda for DSM-V highlights a need to translate basic and clinical neuroscience research findings into a new classification system for all psychiatric disorders based upon pathophysiological and etiological processes. Furthermore, identification of neural system abnormalities in individuals with bipolar disorder is of critical importance for the advance in diagnosis and subsequent treatment of this frequently misdiagnosed disorder, particularly in individuals presenting with depression without a clear history of mania. A first stage toward the identification of biomarkers of bipolar disorder is the examination of functional abnormalities in neural systems directly related to common symptom domains of bipolar disorder that are common to depression and remission, rather than remission or depression specific, and those abnormalities that are specific to bipolar disorder rather than common to unipolar depression. Such common symptom domains include mood instability, linked with impaired emotion processing, and impaired cognitive control processes, linked with cognitive dysfunction, that together may underlie the inability to regulate emotional states in individuals with bipolar disorder. Findings from a small number of studies indicate increased amygdala activity in response to mild happy and fearful facial expressions and decreased DLPFC activity in response to fearful expressions, although no consistent pattern of emotion identification deficits, in remitted individuals with bipolar disorder. There are more consistent findings indicating impaired performance on working memory and attentional tasks in remitted individuals with bipolar disorder. Findings also indicate decreased prefrontal cortical, in particular ventrolateral and dorsal anterior cingulate gyral, activity, but also increased subcortical activity, during attentional task performance in these individuals. Data suggest relative increases in prefrontal cortical activity during attentional task performance in depressed compared with remitted individuals with bipolar disorder. There are limited data examining abnormalities that are common to remitted and depressed individuals with bipolar disorder—or even examining abnormalities that may persist throughout mania—in addition to depression and remission. Very few neuroimaging studies have directly compared bipolar and unipolar populations. Similarly, the relationship between structural and functional neural abnormalities and effects of psychotropic medication upon patterns of abnormal neural responses also remain unclarified in bipolar disorder. Current research should focus upon elucidation of neural system abnormalities that can be identified as biomarkers of bipolar disorder to help improve diagnostic accuracy in individuals in earlier stages of illness using paradigms. Major future goals are then to identify biomarkers that reflect risk for subsequent development of bipolar disorder and biomarkers that enable us to predict treatment response in individuals with the disorder.

References

1. Murray CJL, Lopez AD. The Global Burden of Disease: A Comprehensive Assessment of Mortality and Disability From Disease, Injuries and Risk Factors in 1990 and Projected to 2020. Cambridge, MA: Harvard School of Public Health, Harvard University Press; 1996. On behalf of the World Health Organization and the World Bank.
2. Baldessarini RJ, Tondo L. Suicide risk and treatments for patients with bipolar disorder. JAMA. 2003;290:1517–1519.
3. Wyatt RJ, Henter I. An economic evaluation of manic-depressive illness—1991. Soc Psychiatry Psychiatr Epidemiol. 1995;30:213–219.
4. Bowden CL. Strategies to reduce misdiagnosis of bipolar depression. Psychiatr Serv. 2001;52:51–55.
5. Bowden CL. A different depression: clinical distinctions between bipolar and unipolar depression. J Affect Disord. 2005;84:117–125.
6. Calabrese JR, Hirschfeld RM, Frye MA, Reed ML. Impact of depressive symptoms compared with manic symptoms in bipolar disorder: results of a U.S. community-based sample. J Clin Psychiatry. 2004;65:1499–1504.
7. Ghaemi SN, Hsu DJ, Ko JY, Baldassano CF, Kontos NJ, Goodwin FK. Bipolar spectrum disorder: a pilot study. Psychopathology. 2004;37:222–226.
8. Hirschfeld RM, Lewis L, Vornik LA. Perceptions and impact of bipolar disorder: how far have we really come? Results of the National Depressive and Manic-Depressive Association 2000 survey of individuals with bipolar disorder. J Clin Psychiatry. 2003;64:161–174.
9. Lish JD, Dime-Meenan S, Whybrow PC, Price RA, Hirschfeld RM. The National Depressive and Manic-Depressive Association (DMDA) survey of bipolar members. J Affect Disord. 1994;31:281–294.
10. Manning JS. Bipolar disorder in primary care. J Fam Pract. 2003;3(suppl 1):S6–S9.
11. Charney DS, Barlow DH, Botterton K, et al. Neuroscience research agenda to guide development of a pathophysiologically based classification system. In: Kupfer DJ, First MB, Regier DA, eds. A Research Agenda for DSM-V. Washington DC: American Psychiatric Association; 2002:31–38.

12. Hasler G, Drevets WC, Gould TD, Gottesman II, Manji HK. Toward constructing an endophenotype strategy for bipolar disorders. Biol Psychiatry. 2006;60:93–105.

13. Hasler G, Drevets WC, Manji HK, Charney DS. Discovering endophenotypes for major depression. Neuropsychopharmacology. 2004;29:1765–1781.

14. Phillips ML, Frank E. Redefining bipolar disorder—toward DSM-V. Am J Psychiatry. 2006;163:7.

15. Kraemer HC, Schultz SK, Arndt S. Biomarkers in psychiatry: methodological issues. Am J Geriatr Psychiatry. 2002;10:653–659.

16. Kraemer HC, Gullion CM, Rush AJ, Frank E, Kupfer DJ. Can state and trait variables be disentangled? A methodological framework for psychiatric disorders. Psychiatry Res. 1994;52:55–69.

17. Kupfer DJ. The increasing medical burden in bipolar disorder. JAMA. 2005;293:2528–2530.

18. Swann A. What is bipolar disorder? Am J Psychiatry. 2006;163:177–179.

19. Ochsner KN, Gross JJ. The cognitive control of emotion. Trends Cogn Sci. 2005;9:242–249.

20. Clark L, Kempton MJ, Scarna A, Grasby PM, Goodwin GM. Sustained attention-deficit confirmed in euthymic bipolar disorder but not in first-degree relatives of bipolar patients or euthymic unipolar depression. Biol Psychiatry. 2005;57:183–187.

21. Phillips ML, Drevets WC, Rauch SL, Lane RD. Neurobiology of emotion perception II: implications for major psychiatric disorders. Biol Psychiatry. 2003;54:515–528.

22. Phillips ML, Drevets WC, Rauch SL, Lane RD. Neurobiology of emotion perception I: the neural basis of normal emotion perception. Biol Psychiatry. 2003;54:504–514.

23. Stuss DT, Levine B. Adult clinical neuropsychology: lessons from studies of the frontal lobes. Annu Rev Psychol. 2002;53:401–433.

24. Calder AJ, Lawrence AD, Young AW. Neuropsychology of fear and loathing. Nat Rev Neurosci. 2001;2:352–363.

25. Morris JS, Frith CD, Perrett DI, et al. A differential neural response in the human amygdala to fearful and happy facial expressions. Nature. 1996;383:812–815.

26. Phillips ML, Young AW, Senior C, et al. A specific neural substrate for perceiving facial expressions of disgust. Nature. 1997;389:495–498.

27. Surguladze SA, Brammer MJ, Young AW, et al. A preferential increase in the extrastriate response to signals of danger. Neuroimage. 2003;19:1317–1328.

28. Hariri AR, Mattay VS, Tessitore A, et al. Serotonin transporter genetic variation and the response of the human amygdala. Science. 2002;297:400–403.

29. Monchi O, Petrides M, Petre V, Worsley K, Dagher A. Wisconsin card sorting revisited: distinct neural circuits participating in different stages of the task identified by event-related functional magnetic resonance imaging. J Neurosci. 2001;21:7733–7741.

30. Siegle GJ, Steinhauer SR, Thase ME, Stenger VA, Carter CS. Can't shake that feeling: fMRI assessment of sustained amygdala activity in response to emotional information in depressed individuals. Biol Psychiatry. 2002;51:693–707.

31. Ridderinkhof KR, van den Wildenberg WP, Segalowitz SJ, Carter CS. Neurocognitive mechanisms of cognitive control: the role of prefrontal cortex in action selection, response inhibition, performance monitoring, and reward-based learning. Brain Cogn. 2004;56:129–140.

32. Botvinick MM, Cohen JD, Carter CS. Conflict monitoring and anterior cingulate cortex: an update. Trends Cogn Sci. 2004;8:539–546.
33. Garavan H, Ross TJ, Murphy K, Roche RA, Stein EA. Dissociable executive functions in the dynamic control of behavior: inhibition, error detection, and correction. Neuroimage. 2002;17:1820–1829.
34. Kerns JG, Cohen JD, MacDonald AW III, Cho RY, Stenger VA, Carter CS. Anterior cingulate conflict monitoring and adjustments in control. Science. 2004;303:1023–1026.
35. van Veen V, Holroyd CB, Cohen JD, Stenger VA, Carter CS. Errors without conflict: implications for performance monitoring theories of anterior cingulate cortex. Brain Cogn. 2004;56:267–276.
36. Blumberg HP, Leung HC, Skudlarski P, et al. A functional magnetic resonance imaging study of bipolar disorder: state- and trait-related dysfunction in ventral prefrontal cortices. Arch Gen Psychiatry. 2003;60:601–609.
37. Levesque J, Eugene F, Joanette Y, et al. Neural circuitry underlying voluntary suppression of sadness. Biol Psychiatry. 2003;53:502–510.
38. Phan KL, Fitzgerald DA, Nathan PJ, Moore GJ, Uhde TW, Tancer ME. Neural substrates for voluntary suppression of negative affect: a functional magnetic resonance imaging study. Biol Psychiatry. 2005;57:210–219.
39. Lawrence N, Williams A, Surguladze S, Brammer MJ, Williams SCR, Phillips ML. Subcortical and ventral prefrontal cortical neural responses to facial expressions distinguish patients with bipolar and major depression. Biol Psychiatry. 2004;55:578–587.
40. Yurgelun-Todd DA, Gruber SA, Kanayama G, Killgore WD, Baird AA, Young AD. fMRI during affect discrimination in bipolar affective disorder. Bipolar Disord. 2000;2:237–248.
41. Blumberg HP, Donegan NH, Sanislow CA, et al. Preliminary evidence for medication effects on functional abnormalities in the amygdala and anterior cingulate in bipolar disorder. Psychopharmacology. 2005;183:308–313.
42. Malhi GS, Lagopoulos J, Sachdev PS, Ivanovski B, Shnier R. An emotional Stroop functional MRI study of euthymic bipolar disorder. Bipolar Disord. 2005;7(suppl 5):58–69.
43. Malhi GS, Lagopoulos J, Owen AM, Ivanovski B, Shnier R, Sachdev P. Reduced activation to implicit affect induction in euthymic bipolar patients: an fMRI study. J Affect Disord. 2007;97:109–122.
44. Gruber SA, Rogowska J, Yurgelun-Todd DA. Decreased activation of the anterior cingulate in bipolar patients: an fMRI study. J Affect Disord. 2004;82:191–201.
45. Deckersbach T, Dougherty DD, Savage C, et al. Impaired recruitment of the dorsolateral prefrontal cortex and hippocampus during encoding in bipolar disorder. Biol Psychiatry. 2006;559:138–146.
46. Monks PJ, Thompson JM, Bullmore ET, et al. A functional MRI study of working memory task in euthymic bipolar disorder: evidence for task-specific dysfunction. Bipolar Disord. 2004;6:550–564.
47. Strakowski SM, Adler CM, Holland SK, Mills N, DelBello MP. A preliminary fMRI study of sustained attention in euthymic, unmedicated bipolar disorder. Neuropsychopharmacology. 2004;29:1734–1740.
48. Adler CM, Holland SK, Schmithorst V, Tuchfarber MJ, Strakowski SM. Changes in neuronal activation in patients with bipolar disorder during performance of a working memory task. Bipolar Disord. 2004;6:540–549.

49. Blumberg HP, Martin A, Kaufman J, et al. Frontostriatal abnormalities in adolescents with bipolar disorder: preliminary observations from functional MRI. Am J Psychiatry. 2003;160:1345–1347.

50. Malhi GS, Lagopoulos J, Ward PB, et al. Cognitive generation of affect in bipolar depression: an fMRI study. Eur J Neurosci. 2004;19:741–754.

51. Kruger S, Alda M, Young T, Goldapple K, Parikh S, Mayberg HS. Risk and resilience markers in bipolar disorder: brain responses to emotional challenge in bipolar patients and their healthy siblings. Am J Psychiatry. 2006;163:257–264.

52. Kruger S, Seminowicz D, Goldapple K, Kennedy SH, Mayberg HS. State and trait influences on mood regulation in bipolar disorder: blood flow differences with an acute mood challenge. Biol Psychiatry. 2003;54:1274–1283.

53. Chen C-H, Lennox B, Jacob R, et al. Explicit and implicit facial affect recognition in manic and depressed states of bipolar disorder: a functional magnetic resonance imaging study. Biol Psychiatry. 2005;59:31–39.

54. Drevets WC, Price JL, Bardgett ME, Reich T, Todd RD, Raichle ME. Glucose metabolism in the amygdala in depression: relationship to diagnostic subtype and plasma cortisol levels. Pharmacol Biochem Behav. 2002;71:431–447.

55. Ketter TA, Kimbrell TA, George MS, et al. Effects of mood and subtype on cerebral glucose metabolism in treatment-resistant bipolar disorder. Biol Psychiatry. 2001;49:97–109.

56. Kronhaus DM, Lawrence N, Williams AM, et al. The ventral prefrontal cortex in bipolar disorder: distinguishing trait and depression-related abnormalities. Bipolar Disord. 2006;8:28–39.

57. Altshuler LL, Bookheimer SY, Townsend J, et al. Blunted activation in orbitofrontal cortex during mania: a functional magnetic resonance imaging study. Biol Psychiatry. 2005;58:763–769.

58. Lennox BR, Jacob R, Calder AJ, Lupson V, Bullmore ET. Behavioural and neurocognitive responses to sad facial affect are attenuated in patients with mania. Psychol Med. 2004;34:795–802.

59. Malhi GS, Lagopoulos J, Sachdev P, Mitchell PB, Ivanovski B, Parker GB. Cognitive generation of affect in hypomania: an fMRI study. Bipolar Disord. 2004;6:271–285.

60. Blumberg HP, Stern E, Martinez D, et al. Increased anterior cingulate and caudate activity in bipolar mania. Biol Psychiatry. 2000;48:1045–1052.

61. Caligiuri MP, Brown GG, Meloy MJ, et al. An fMRI study of affective state and medication on cortical and subcortical brain regions during motor performance in bipolar disorder. Psychiatry Res. 2003;123:171–182.

62. Altshuler L, Bookheimer S, Proenza MA, et al. Increased amygdala activation during mania: a functional magnetic resonance imaging study. Am J Psychiatry. 2005;162:1211–1213.

63. Blumberg HP, Stern E, Ricketts S, et al. Rostral and orbital prefrontal cortex dysfunction in the manic state of bipolar disorder. Am J Psychiatry. 1999;156:1986–1988.

64. Elliott R, Ogilvie A, Rubinsztein JS, Calderon G, Dolan RJ, Sahakian BJ. Abnormal ventral frontal response during performance of an affective go/no go task in patients with mania. Biol Psychiatry. 2004;55:1163–1170.

65. Rubinsztein JS, Fletcher PC, Rogers RD, et al. Decision-making in mania: a PET study. Brain. 2001;124(pt 12): 2550–2563.

66. Baxter LR Jr, Schwartz JM, Phelps ME, et al. Reduction of prefrontal cortex glucose metabolism common to three types of depression. Arch Gen Psychiatry. 1989;46:243–250.
67. Mayberg HS, Brannan SK, Tekell JL, et al. Regional metabolic effects of fluoxetine in major depression: serial changes and relationship to clinical response. Biol Psychiatry. 2000;48:830–843.
68. Brody AL, Saxena S, Stoessel P, et al. Regional brain metabolic changes in patients with major depression treated with either paroxetine or interpersonal therapy: preliminary findings. Arch Gen Psychiatry. 2001;58:631–640.
69. Martin SD, Martin E, Rai SS, Richardson MA, Royall R. Brain blood flow changes in depressed patients treated with interpersonal psychotherapy or venlafaxine hydrochloride: preliminary findings. Arch Gen Psychiatry. 2001;58:641–648.
701. Goldapple K, Segal Z, Garson C, et al. Modulation of cortical-limbic pathways in major depression: treatment-specific effects of cognitive behavior therapy. Arch Gen Psychiatry. 2004;6:34–41.
71. Kennedy SH, Evans KR, Kruger S, et al. Changes in regional brain glucose metabolism measured with positron emission tomography after paroxetine treatment of major depression. Am J Psychiatry. 2001;158:899–905.
72. Goodwin GM, Austin MP, Dougall N, et al. State changes in brain activity shown by the uptake of 99mTc-exametazime with single photon emission tomography in major depression before and after treatment. J Affect Disord. 1993;29:243–253.
73. Holthoff VA, Beuthien-Baumann B, Zundorf G, et al. Changes in brain metabolism associated with remission in unipolar major depression. Acta Psychiatr Scand. 2004;110:184–194.
74. Tutus A, Simsek A, Sofuoglu S, et al. Changes in regional cerebral blood flow demonstrated by single photon emission computed tomography in depressive disorders: comparison of unipolar vs. bipolar subtypes. Psychiatry Res. 1998;83:169–177.
75. Vlassenko A, Sheline YI, Fischer K, Mintun MA. Cerebral perfusion response to successful treatment of depression with different serotoninergic agents. J Neuropsychiatry Clin Neurosci. 2004;16:360–363.
76. Martinot JL, Hardy P, Feline A. Left prefrontal glucose hypometabolism in the depressed state: a confirmation. Am J Psychiatry. 1990;147:1313–1317.
77. Saxena S, Brody AL, Ho ML, et al. Differential cerebral metabolic changes with paroxetine treatment of obsessive-compulsive disorder vs major depression. Arch Gen Psychiatry. 2002;59:250–261.
78. Kimbrell TA, Ketter TA, George MS, et al. Regional cerebral glucose utilization in patients with a range of severities of unipolar depression. Biol Psychiatry. 2002;51:237–252.
79. Fu CH, Williams SC, Cleare AJ, et al. Attenuation of the neural response to sad faces in major depression by antidepressant treatment: a prospective, event-related functional magnetic resonance imaging study. Arch Gen Psychiatry. 2004;61:877–889.
80. Sheline YI, Barch DM, Donnelly JM, Ollinger JM, Snyder AZ, Mintun MA. Increased amygdala response to masked emotional faces in depressed subjects resolves with antidepressant treatment: an fMRI study. Biol Psychiatry. 2001;50:651–658.

81. Surguladze S, Brammer M, Keedwell P, et al. A differential pattern of neural response towards sad versus happy facial expressions in major depressive disorder. Biol Psychiatry. 2005;57:201–209.

82. Liotti M, Mayberg HS, McGinnis S, Brannan SL, Jerabek P. Unmasking disease-specific cerebral blood flow abnormalities: mood challenge in patients with remitted unipolar depression. Am J Psychiatry. 2002;159:1830–1840.

83. Elliott R, Baker SC, Rogers RD, et al. Prefrontal dysfunction in depressed patients performing a complex planning task: a study using positron emission tomography. Psychol Med. 1997;27:931–942.

84. Goethals I, Audenaert K, Jacobs F, et al. Blunted prefrontal perfusion in depressed patients performing the Tower of London task. Psychiatry Res. 2005;139:31–40.

85. Okada G, Okamoto Y, Morinobu S, Yamawaki S, Yokota N. Attenuated left prefrontal activation during a verbal fluency task in patients with depression. Neuropsychobiology. 2003;47:21–26.

86. Davidson RJ, Irwin W, Anderle MJ, Kalin NH. The neural substrates of affective processing in depressed patients treated with venlafaxine. Am J Psychiatry. 2003;160:64–75.

87. Price JL. Comparative aspects of amygdala connectivity. Ann N Y Acad Sci. 2003;985:50–58.

88. Altshuler LL, Bartzokis G, Grieder T, Curran J, Mintz J. Amygdala enlargement in bipolar disorder and hippocampal reduction in schizophrenia: an MRI study demonstrating neuroanatomic specificity. Arch Gen Psychiatry. 1998;55:663–664.

89. Altshuler LL, Bartzokis G, Grieder T, et al. An MRI study of temporal lobe structures in men with bipolar disorder or schizophrenia. Biol Psychiatry. 2000;48:147–162.

90. Brambilla P, Harenski K, Nicoletti M, et al. MRI investigation of temporal lobe structures in bipolar patients. J Psychiatr Res. 2003;37:287–295.

91. Frangou S. The Maudsley bipolar disorder project. Epilepsia. 2005;46(suppl 4):19–25.

92. Strakowski SM, DelBello MP, Sax KW, et al. Brain magnetic resonance imaging of structural abnormalities in bipolar disorder. Arch Gen Psychiatry. 1999;56:254–260.

93. Benabarre A, Vieta E, Martinez-Aran A, et al. The somatics of psyche: structural neuromorphometry of bipolar disorder. Psychother Psychosom. 2002;71:180–189.

94. Blumberg HP, Kaufman J, Martin A, et al. Amygdala and hippocampal volumes in adolescents and adults with bipolar disorder. Arch Gen Psychiatry. 2003;60:1201–1208.

95. Blumberg HP, Fredericks C, Wang F, et al. Preliminary evidence for persistent abnormalities in amygdala volumes in adolescents and young adults with bipolar disorder. Bipolar Disord. 2005;7:570–576.

96. Chang K, Karchemskiy A, Barnea-Goraly N, Garrett A, Simeonova DI, Reiss A. Reduced amygdalar gray matter volume in familial pediatric bipolar disorder. J Am Acad Child Adolesc Psychiatry. 2005;44:565–573.

97. Chen BK, Sassi R, Axelson D, et al. Cross-sectional study of abnormal amygdala development in adolescents and young adults with bipolar disorder. Biol Psychiatry. 2004;56:399–405.

98. DelBello MP, Zimmerman ME, Mills NP, Getz GE, Strakowski SM. Magnetic resonance imaging analysis of amygdala and other subcortical brain regions in adolescents with bipolar disorder. Bipolar Disord. 2004;6:43–52.

99. Dickstein DP, Milham MP, Nugent AC, et al. Frontotemporal alterations in pediatric bipolar disorder: results of a voxel-based morphometry study. Arch Gen Psychiatry. 2005;62:734–741.

100. Aylward EH, Roberts-Twillie JV, Barta PE, et al. Basal ganglia volumes and white matter hyperintensities in patients with bipolar disorder. Am J Psychiatry. 1994;151:687–693.

101. McIntosh AM, Job DE, Moorhead TW, et al. Voxel-based morphometry of patients with schizophrenia or bipolar disorder and their unaffected relatives. Biol Psychiatry. 2004;56:544–552.

102. Hastings RS, Parsey RV, Oquendo MA, Arango V, Mann JJ. Volumetric analysis of the prefrontal cortex, amygdala, and hippocampus in major depression. Neuropsychopharmacology. 2004;29:952–959.

103. Sheline YI, Gado MH, Kraemer HC. Untreated depression and hippocampal volume loss. Am J Psychiatry. 2003;160:1516–1518.

104. Siegle GJ, Konecky RO, Thase ME, Carter CS. Relationships between amygdala volume and activity during emotional information processing tasks in depressed and never-depressed individuals: an fMRI investigation. Ann NY Acad Sci. 2003;985:481–484.

105. Bruno SD, Barker GJ, Cercignani M, Symms M, Ron MA. A study of bipolar disorder using magnetization transfer imaging and voxel-based morphometry. Brain. 2004;127:2433–2440.

106. Lochhead RA, Parsey RV, Oquendo MA, Mann JJ. Regional brain gray matter volume differences in patients with bipolar disorder as assessed by optimized voxel-based morphometry. Biol Psychiatry. 2004;55:1154–1162.

107. Lyoo IK, Kim MJ, Stoll AL, et al. Frontal lobe gray matter density decreases in bipolar I disorder. Biol Psychiatry. 2004;55:648–651.

108. Sassi RB, Brambilla P, Hatch JP, et al. Reduced left anterior cingulate volumes in untreated bipolar patients. Biol Psychiatry. 2004;56:467–475.

109. Lopez-Larson MP, DelBello MP, Zimmerman ME, Schwiers ML, Strakowski SM. Regional prefrontal gray and white matter abnormalities in bipolar disorder. Biol Psychiatry. 2002;52:93–100.

110. Sax KW, Strakowski SM, Zimmerman ME, DelBello MP, Keck PE Jr, Hawkins JM. Frontosubcortical neuroanatomy and the continuous performance test in mania. Am J Psychiatry. 1999;156:139–141.

111. Sharma V, Menon R, Carr TJ, Densmore M, Mazmanian D, Williamson PC. An MRI study of subgenual prefrontal cortex in patients with familial and non-familial bipolar I disorder. J Affect Disord. 2003;77:167–171.

112. Adler CM, Holland SK, Schmithorst V, et al. Abnormal frontal white matter tracts in bipolar disorder: a diffusion tensor imaging study. Bipolar Disord. 2004;20:197–203.

113. Nugent AC, Milham MP, Bain EE, et al. Cortical abnormalities in bipolar disorder investigated with MRI and voxel-based morphometry. Neuroimage. 2006;30:485–497.

114. Brambilla P, Nicoletti MA, Harenski K, et al. Anatomical MRI study of subgenual prefrontal cortex in bipolar and unipolar subjects. Neuropsychopharmacology. 2002;27:792–799.

115. Sanches M, Sassi RB, Axelson D, et al. Subgenual prefrontal cortex of child and adolescent bipolar patients: a morphometric magnetic resonance imaging study. Psychiatry Res. 2005;138:43–49.
116. Caetano SC, Kaur S, Brambilla P, et al. Smaller cingulate volumes in unipolar depressed patients. Biol Psychiatry. 2004;59:702–706.
117. Drevets WC, Price JL, Simpson JR Jr, et al. Subgenual prefrontal cortex abnormalities in mood disorders. Nature. 1997;386:824–827.
118. Kanner AM. Structural MRI changes of the brain in depression. Clin EEG Neurosci. 2004;35:46–52.
119. Lavretsky H, Kurbanyan K, Ballmaier M, Mintz J, Toga A, Kumar A. Sex differences in brain structure in geriatric depression. Am J Geriatr Psychiatry. 2004;12:653–657.
120. Strakowski SM, Delbello MP, Adler CM. The functional neuroanatomy of bipolar disorder: a review of neuroimaging findings. Mol Psychiatry. 2005;10:105–116.
121. McDonald C, Zanelli J, Rabe-Hesketh S, et al. Meta-analysis of magnetic resonance imaging brain morphometry studies in bipolar disorder. Biol Psychiatry. 2004;56:411–417.
122. Paulus MP, Feinstein JS, Castillo G, Simmons AN, Stein MB. Dose-dependent decrease of activation in bilateral amygdala and insula by lorazepam during emotion processing. Arch Gen Psychiatry. 2005;62:282–288.
123. Del-Ben CM, Deakin JF, McKie S, et al. The effect of citalopram pretreatment on neuronal responses to neuropsychological tasks in normal volunteers: an FMRI study. Neuropsychopharmacology. 2005;30:1724–1734.
124. Takahashi H, Yahata N, Koeda M, et al. Effects of dopaminergic and serotonergic manipulation on emotional processing: a pharmacological fMRI study. Neuroimage. 2005;27:991–1001.
125. Harmer CJ, Mackay CE, Rein CB, Cowen PJ, Goodwin GM. Antidepressant drug treatment modifies the neural processing of nonconscious threat cues. Biol Psychiatry. 2006;59:816–821.
126. Kemp AH, Gray MA, Silberstein RB, Armstrong SM, Nathan PJ. Augmentation of serotonin enhances pleasant and suppresses unpleasant cortical electrophysiological responses to visual emotional stimuli in humans. Neuroimage. 2004;22:1084–1096.
127. Strakowski SM, Adler CM, Holland SK, Mills NP, DelBello MP, Eliassen JC. Abnormal FMRI brain activation in euthymic bipolar disorder patients during a counting Stroop interference task. Am J Psychiatry. 2005;162:1697–1705.
128. Manji HK, Drevets WC, Charney DS. The cellular neurobiology of depression. Nat Med. 2001;7:541–547.
129. Vieta E, Gasto C, Otero A, Nieto E, Vallejo J. Differential features between bipolar I and bipolar II disorder. Compr Psychiatry. 1997;38:98–101.
130. Torrent C, Martinez-Aran A, Daban C, et al. Cognitive impairment in bipolar II disorder. Br J Psychiatry. 2006;189:254–259.
131. McDonald C, Bullmore ET, Sham PC, et al. Association of genetic risks for schizophrenia and bipolar disorder with specific and generic brain structural endophenotypes. Arch Gen Psychiatry. 2004;61:974–984.
132. Cecil KM, DelBello MP, Sellars MC, Strakowski SM. Proton magnetic resonance spectroscopy of the frontal lobe and cerebellar vermis in children with a mood disorder and a familial risk for bipolar disorders. J Child Adolesc Psychopharmacol. 2003;13:545–555.

11

THE NEUROPHARMACOLOGY OF PSYCHOSIS

Carol A. Tamminga, M.D.
John M. Davis, M.D.

This chapter reviews the drug treatments for psychotic illnesses for the purpose of considering whether "psychosis" is a more cohesive biological entity and illness category than the *Diagnostic and Statistical Manual of Mental Disorders,* 4th Edition (DSM-IV)[1] diagnostic entities that have psychosis as one of their symptoms. Because schizophrenia (SZ) and bipolar-1 disorder (BP-1) are the two diagnoses that have the most similar phenotypes, we have examined the pharmacology of these two diagnoses in detail, as illustrative of psychotic disorders. Scientists have often taken the mechanism of action of antipsychotic drugs (APDs) as a clue to the pathological mechanisms of psychosis itself. It is a logical postulate from this idea that psychotic symptoms, even across diagnoses, might be mechanistically related. Do commonalities in the treatment response of psychotic disorders suggest that psychotic illnesses should be considered dimensionally instead of diagnostically? The chapter is one of a series of reviews in this monograph based on different perspectives (e.g., phenomenology, imaging, clinical genetics, molecular analysis) intended to address this same question: what are the data to support the consideration of the dimension of psychosis as a diagnostic entity?

Reprinted with permission from Tamminga CA, Davis JM. "The Neuropharmacology of Psychosis." *Schizophrenia Bulletin* 2007; 33: 937–946.

We think that the following anecdote illustrates problems with diagnostic nomenclature. Dr. William Sargent was a leading British psychiatrist noted for his enthusiasm for drug treatment in mental disorders and his criticisms of psychoanalysis. He visited the National Institute of Mental Health in 1964. At the same time, a distinguished American psychoanalyst, Dexter Bullard, also visited. He was an enthusiast of psychoanalytic treatment and opposed to the use of medications for mental illness. Both distinguished psychiatrists jointly interviewed six patients on a clinical unit and then retired for an informal discussion. One remarked that it was obvious that three of the patients had one disorder and three had a different disorder. The other agreed exactly and remarked that it was surprising that they could agree on anything. It turned out that they were in agreement on which three individuals had one disorder and which three had the other disorder but were in disagreement about what the disorders were. Dr. Sargent felt that three patients had depression (a biological disease) and three patients had hysteria with secondary depression (a psychoneurotic disorder). Dr. Bullard thought that the first three patients had SZ and the second three patients had depression. The first three patients in modern DSM-IV categorization would be diagnosed as having severe endogenous psychotic depression. We use this anecdote to raise the question of whether diagnostic categorization could be usefully augmented by dimensional considerations.

On a more general level, in the 1950s and early 1960s, there was substantial disagreement on diagnosis between British and American psychiatrists. In the United States, mania was uncommonly diagnosed and, if it was diagnosed, it was generally applied to a euphoric mania without psychotic features. SZ was very broadly diagnosed in the United States. Mania with psychosis was more typically diagnosed in the United Kingdom. Since then, consensus diagnoses based on phenomenology and guided by accepted criteria have aided our ability to apply similar labels to a given clinical phenomenon. This system has not served to foster (and may have hindered) the identification of mechanisms of the mental illnesses and new treatment directions.

Dimensional Aspects of Diagnoses

In this chapter, we will review and discuss the neuropharmacology of psychotic illnesses, particularly SZ and BP-1. We have selected these two diagnoses as illustrative among the psychoses because of their phenomenological similarities. We will review their common and distinctive pharmacological characteristics. In time, this perspective could be used to refine clinical targets for treatment development for psychosis. We will speculate on the possibility of a common mechanism or a common "final pathway" for the psychoses. Whether this should be the basis of a new dimensional categorization among psychotic illnesses is a related question, but one for which we have little pertinent data.

APDs are widely used and effective in the treatment of psychosis across many psychotic diagnostic classifications, including such diagnoses as SZ, bipolar disorder (BD), psychotic depression (major depressive disorder), dementia, dopamine agonist–induced psychoses, various organic psychoses, and certain aggressive or self-injury behavior in the mentally retarded. Psychosis is a pathological mental state characterized by the abnormal interpretation, organization, and/or use of cognitive stimuli, those generated internally and encountered externally. It includes an inability to distinguish between real and not real stimuli. Gardner, Baldessarini, and Waraich[2] described the use of APDs for psychosis:

> Antipsychotic drugs are useful for treating a range of severe psychiatric disorders. Applications include the short-term treatment of acute psychotic, manic and psychotic-depressive disorders as well as agitated states in delirium and dementia and the long-term treatment of chronic psychotic disorders, including schizophrenia, schizoaffective disorder and delusional disorders.

It is common within diagnostic categories to describe symptoms phenomenologically, using domains. Domains are groups of symptoms that resemble each other and correlate with each other over disease course and across individuals. This categorization was originally done to aid diagnostic classification. But more recently, scientists have explored its usefulness in identifying clinical targets for drug development.[3] A recent example of the use of a domain orientation in augmenting drug development has been the focus on cognition in SZ. The emphasis on cognition developed because of the realization that psychosis in SZ is reasonably well treated with first- and second-generation APDs; however, the residual impairments in cognition impede full psychosocial recovery. This realization suggested an emphasis on treatment development for cognition in SZ, a project led by the Measurement and Treatment Research to Improve Cognition in Schizophrenia (MATRICS) group and now represented by Treatment Units for Research on Neurocognition and Schizophrenia (TURNS).[4] The SZ domains commonly include psychosis, cognitive dysfunction, and negative symptoms. Within SZ, these domains developed from factor analytic studies of large patient data sets (reviewed in Carpenter and Buchanan[5]). These data sets established that the domains are independent and, therefore, could have their own mechanisms. It is only logical to speculate about whether similar domains across diagnostic categories share biological mechanisms and clinical prognosis, especially if their pharmacology is similar. In parallel, BD could be said to include some similar and some unique symptom domains: psychosis, cognitive dysfunction, and mood dysregulation with mania and depression. Less is known about negative symptoms in bipolar illness. However, the extent to which the domains in SZ and BP-1 with similar names are in fact the same construct is not known. For example, is the psychosis domain across SZ and BP-1 the same clinically, genetically, and mechanistically, and do both domains show the same treatment response?

Psychiatric practice and controlled studies in specific diagnostic groups suggest that the psychotic symptom domain is treated with similar medications across diagnoses, and we know that psychosis responds therapeutically to those treatments. Nonetheless, these are clinical observations drawn from clinical practice, not results from controlled clinical trials inclusive of multiple diagnoses. Multiple questions exist, including whether or not the psychotic symptoms overlap descriptively (rated with the same scale), whether they respond on the same time course, and the extent to which associated domains are also treated. It is important to note that not all symptom domains currently have effective treatments. Within the diagnosis of SZ, for example, effective treatments exist primarily for psychosis, while neither cognitive deficits nor core negative symptoms have demonstrated drug treatments.[6]

In this chapter, we will review therapeutic data from the fields of SZ and BP-1 research and examine the extent to which psychosis is treated similarly across these two diagnoses. We will do this as an example of studying domain treatment across diagnoses. We will review data on efficacy and effectiveness of APDs in each diagnosis, of side effect patterns, of their influence on co-occurring symptoms and on the postulated mechanisms of APD action. It is important to notice before starting that the data required to directly answer the questions raised in this section have not been collected, i.e., data where the same set of drugs are compared across diagnoses in the same study with parallel methodologies. So, this review will not be able to arrive at a final answer, only the commonalities in clinical responses.

Efficacy of APDs in Schizophrenia

In clinical practice, the treatment of psychosis in SZ is approached using either the second- or the first-generation APDs.[7] These drugs are used for acute treatment and for maintenance. Deciding on the specific APD among the candidates is characteristically made on an individual basis, taking drug action and side effects into consideration. There is excellent evidence that both first-generation antipsychotics (FGAs) and second-generation antipsychotics (SGAs) substantially benefit SZ better than placebo alone based on more than 30 recent double-blind studies[8] and consistent with a much larger number of controlled studies done more than 20 years ago (reviewed in Davis[9]). There are also a number of comparisons of second-generation drugs versus first-generation drugs[10–14] and a smaller number of comparisons among second-generation drugs where one of the comparators was olanzapine.[10] In Table 11–1, we show a summary of the effect sizes of studies contrasting FGAs with SGAs. It is only clozapine that shows moderate to large effect size differences from FGAs on clinical outcome. Olanzapine and risperidone show low to moderate effect size differences from FGAs, but not in every study. Below, we discuss the results of several recent studies. These data are interpreted differently by various observers.

TABLE 11–1. Drug efficacy in effect size units

Comparator	Davis FGA[11]	Cochrane FGA[11]	Geddes FGA[11]	Leucht FGA[12,13]	Leucht low-potency FGA[13]	CATIE-1[a] FGA[15]	CATIE-T[b] FGA[17]	CATIE-Eff[b] FGA[16]
Clozapine	0.49	0.38	0.66		0.15			1.12
Olanzapine	0.21	0.27	0.22	0.08	0.22	0.32	0.32	0.32
Risperidone	0.25	0.09	0.16	0.17	0.29	-0.04	0.22	0.15
Amisulpride	0.29		0.34	0.23	-0.07			
Zotepine	0.15	0.40			0.17			
Quetiapine	-0.10	-0.10	0.03	-0.10	0.13	-0.09	-0.01	0.15
Ziprasidone	-0.03					0.09	0.09	
Aripiprazole	0.00							
Sertindole	0.03		-0.06	-0.06				
Remoxipride	-0.09				-0.05			

Note. CATIE-1 = Clinical Antipsychotic Trials of Intervention Effectiveness Study, Phase 1; CATIE-Eff = Clinical Antipsychotic Trials of Intervention Effectiveness Study, Efficacy; CATIE-T = Clinical Antipsychotic Trials of Intervention Effectiveness Study, Tolerability; FGA = first-generation antipsychotics; SGA = second-generation antipsychotics.

[a] Duration of successful treatment of CATIE-1 is similar to efficacy. We calculated the effect size by using the *P* values under the column label perphenazine and the sample size of this drug and of the SGAs without tardive dyskinesia. Because CATIE-T and Catie-Eff did not have a typical arm, we expressed the effect size of each of the other drugs based on its difference from olanzapine, and assigned olanzapine the same effect size as CATIE-1. This is only an approximation but does not put all effect sizes as a comparison of typical.

[b] Drug efficacy in effect size units of SGAs compared against FGAs like haloperidol. A "0.00" would indicate no difference; a positive number indicates that the second-generation drug is more efficacious.

In SZ, one of the most recent, naturalistic studies of SGAs in SZ is the Clinical Antipsychotic Trials of Intervention Effectiveness (CATIE) study.[15] The large patient sample (*N*= 1,493) makes these data important, and the comparison of olanzapine, risperidone, quetiapine, ziprasidone, and perphenazine makes the data broadly relevant. The naturalistic design makes the data more representative, while the methodology is less controlled. In the CATIE study, there were subsequent treatment opportunities after discontinuing, so that "discontinuation" could more aptly be called "switching." In this context, the study discontinuation rate was surprisingly high: overall, 74% of the volunteers discontinued phase 1 before 18 months, with 64% discontinuing olanzapine; 75%, perphenazine; 82%, quetiapine; 74%, risperidone; and 79%, ziprasidone. Olanzapine was the most effective drug in phase 1 as measured by "rate of discontinuation" (which was the study's primary outcome measure) and on several of the secondary efficacy outcomes, but it also was associated with the highest weight gain and greatest increases in metabolic measures.

In the phase 2 CATIE study, where volunteers terminated phase 1 for "ineffectiveness," 99 volunteers were tested with clozapine compared with olanzapine, risperidone, or quetiapine. The results of this comparison showed a large effectiveness advantage for clozapine,[16] with its time-to-discontinuation nearly three times longer than time-to-discontinuation with the other SGAs. In the phase 2 CATIE study, where volunteers terminated phase 1 for "intolerable side effects," 444 volunteers were tested with olanzapine, risperidone, quetiapine, or ziprasidone. Of these treatments, olanzapine and risperidone had equivalent effectiveness, and both were better than quetiapine or ziprasidone by significant but modest margins.[17]

Aripiprazole, given its later entrance into the APD market, has fewer studies available, especially nonsponsor studies. In this context, its registration studies show a significant antipsychotic action of aripiprazole against placebo and of equivalent magnitude with comparator drugs.[18–21] El-Sayeh and Morganti[22] in a Cochrane Database Systematic Review concluded that aripiprazole has equal efficacy to FGAs and SGAs with some benefits in side effect profile (lower akathisia, less prolactin elevations, and QT_c prolongation). Later studies demonstrated that aripiprazole shows equal efficacy to olanzapine in chronic stable patient volunteers as well as in those with acute relapse,[23] with aripiprazole showing a better safety profile with respect to motor and to metabolic side effects.

Clinical practice for maintenance of antipsychotic effect in SZ includes the chronic administration of APDs for the lifelong duration of illness.[7] Those studies that have tested the need for maintenance of APDs in early psychosis have characteristically been unsuccessful because of the high rate of relapse once psychosis is manifest. Predictors for relapse exist.[24–26] In early SZ, haloperidol and olanzapine were found to have comparable efficacy on symptom reduction; however, olanzapine showed an advantage on two secondary measures: time to study discontinuation and remission rates.[27,28]

A 1-year comparison of haloperidol, olanzapine, and risperidone showed a greater cognitive benefit of the two SGAs on several aspects of cognitive performance compared with haloperidol; the two SGAs were not different from each other.[28] Harvey et al[29] compared quetiapine and risperidone on cognitive outcomes in a large acute treatment study that included measures of social cognition. They found that both SGA treatments, though studied only for 8 weeks, improved some domains of cognitive dysfunction; they assessed social cognition in parallel and correlated changes in social cognition with neuropsychological gains. Lack of efficacy with traditional or new APDs prompts the use of clozapine in SZ.[30]

Monotherapy with mood stabilizers (lithium, the carbamazepines, valproate, lamotrigine) or antidepressants (tricyclic, monoamine oxidase inhibitor, serotonin uptake inhibitors, or other antidepressants) or the benzodiazepines do not improve psychosis in SZ, but these drugs are often used along with APDs to treat affective symptoms of the illness. However, old as well as recent data show no benefits to outcome for concomitant psychotropic medications in chronic SZ and challenge this aspect of clinical practice.[31] We know of no evidence that lithium, carbamazepine, oxcarbazepine, or valproate produce an additional long-term benefit in most schizophrenic patients. There is some evidence that schizophrenic patients who seem to have recurrent episodes of depression superimposed on top of their SZ may benefit from antidepressants. For space reasons, we cannot review the many control studies of polypharmacy and the very large anecdotal literature.

Efficacy of APDs in BP-1 Psychosis

Lithium, divalproate, or the carbamazepines were traditionally used to treat BP-1. Once SGAs became available (in contrast to the FGAs whose motor side effects in BD were limiting), the SGAs were broadly applied to BD psychosis. APD treatment has been shown to be just as effective in the treatment of active BP-1 psychosis as mood stabilizers.[27,32–34] It is possible that APDs could have inherent mood-stabilizing properties, given the effectiveness of some of the SGAs in maintenance.

The efficacy of lithium in BD mania was discovered in 1949; the drug was approved by the U.S. Food and Drug Administration (FDA) for this indication in 1970. The discovery of lithium predated the discovery of the antipsychotic action of chlorpromazine in 1953. Chlorpromazine was found effective for acute mania also in the early 1950s. It was FDA approved for the same indication in 1973. In Europe, FGAs were used to treat acute episodes of mania, with mood stabilizers reserved for long-term maintenance. It should not be surprising that if FGAs benefit acute mania, SGAs would also do so. This has been demonstrated in several studies.[35] All the SGAs have been approved for the treatment of acute mania in BD, but with cautions regarding side effects.[36,37] Olanzapine was the first of the SGAs to be approved in 2000, and the other SGAs followed quickly, with risperidone approval in 2003 and quetiapine, ziprasidone, and aripiprazole in 2004.[34] Although in 2000, clinicians were cautious about accepting SGAs as antimanic,[38] the literature burgeoned in the following decade, convincing clinicians of their efficacy.[39]

Efficacy is no longer doubted for the treatment of an acute manic episode in BD. However, the tolerability of the APDs in BD is always questioned,[40] especially the FGAs, which have a high incidence of parkinsonism and tardive dyskinesia (higher in affective than in nonaffective patients[41]). In a medication utilization study done in 2004, the proportion of a large ($n=155$) first-admission cohort with BP-1 receiving APDs at hospitalization discharge was 80%, compared with 52.3% who received antimanic drugs. After 1 year, however, 44.6% of the BP-1 cohort were medication free, with only 19.4% taking APDs and 38.8% taking antimanics.[42] American Psychiatric Association treatment guidelines acknowledge the efficacy of SGAs in BD, in acute mania with psychosis, and even in maintenance treatment for either persistent psychosis or psychosis prophylaxis.[33] In acute mania, however, mood stabilizers are also effective antimanic agents,[43] even though 25%–67% of all acute manic episodes include delusions and 13%–40% include hallucinations. With mood stabilizer monotherapy, many patients achieve syndromal remission without functional remission.[44] With SGA treatment, affective psychosis achieves higher rates of both syndromal and functional recovery than do nonaffective psychoses.[45]

There is evidence that a combination of SGAs with mood stabilizers results in a better response than either treatment alone in BP-1. Schatzberg[46] emphasized that drugs for mood disorders have distinct actions on different BD symptoms, dependent on their mechanism of pharmacological action; APDs decrease psychosis, lithium and valproate stabilize mood dysregulation, and lamotrigine affects depression. With combination treatment using an SGA and mood stabilizer, relapse rates are reduced, efficacy increased, and time to clinical effectiveness reduced.[46] Several reviews[32,47] have emphasized safety and tolerability in selecting a treatment for BP-1 because compliance is critical in maintaining positive drug effect.

APD treatments benefit psychosis in both SZ and BD, including in psychotic and nonpsychotic mania. This leads us to conclude that psychosis in these two categories responds therapeutically to APDs. Yet these clinical observations provide little certainty of how the outcomes in both diagnoses would compare if responses were tested in a single experiment using similar rating scales; whether treatment responses would be the same across the diagnoses still has to be demonstrated. A firm hypothesis that similar psychosis mechanisms operate across disease diagnoses would require careful, controlled experiments with relevant disease categories represented in the study populations.

Treatment of Other Affective Dimensions

The two previous sections reviewed the APD treatments for SZ and BP-1 in detail. There are similar clinical literatures available for other psychotic disorders as well, some of which are included in other chapters in this book. APDs in general are used to treat psychotic symptoms no matter what the diagnosis. In contrast to antipsychotics, drugs for affective disorders are somewhat less specific. Before the antipsychotic, antidepressant, and mood stabilizer drugs were discovered, electroconvulsive therapy (ECT) was widely used in psychiatry. It produced no lasting important benefit in most schizophrenic patients, although it was dramatically effective in both mania and depression.[48] A small group of schizophrenic patients were benefited by ECT, at least in the short term. Lamotrigine has not been shown to be an effective treatment in acute episodes of mania or in the prevention of recurrences of the manic phase.[49,50] Aripiprazole maintenance prevents recurrence of the mania but not the depressive relapse. Lithium is effective in treating acute manic attack; it prevents the recurrence of both manic and depressive episodes during long-term maintenance treatment.[51,52] Lithium is effective in preventing suicide in bipolar disease.[51–53] It does a marginally better job of preventing the recurrence of mania rather than depression, but these are small differences. The effect of lithium compared with placebo in preventing mania or depression is substantial and significant. Lithium is a weak antidepressant for the acute episode of depression but does prevent the recurrence of recurrent unipolar depression.[51,52]

An important issue in affective illness is to distinguish between drug efficacy for acute phases of a manic or depressive episode and the prevention of recurrences of manic and depressive episodes. Some SGAs are active on all phases,[54,55] but many have not been studied in all illness phases. Olanzapine/fluoxetine combination and quetiapine are useful in acute bipolar depression.[56–61] We would caution against the assumption that because one member of a class of drugs has a beneficial effect in a given phase other members of the class will show a beneficial effect. Efficacy in distinct illness phases needs to be demonstrated. For example, it was once assumed that anticonvulsants would treat manic-depressive disease; gabapentin was widely used for this reason. Unfortunately, controlled studies found that gabapentin failed to have efficacy in manic-depressive disease.[62] In psychotic depression, both antipsychotics and antidepressants are needed for the successful treatment. Antipsychotics benefits the psychoses and antidepressants the depression.

One clinically important question in all psychotic illnesses is the extent to which an effective drug in one domain will influence symptoms in another domain. This question becomes especially relevant when considering whether mood stabilizer treatment in psychotic mania affects just mood regulation or treats the psychotic symptoms as well. Because controlled studies show efficacy for both mood stabilizers and APDs in BP-1, clinical practice is confirmed. If the psychosis is not primary, but secondary to mood instability, then psychosis treatment could be effective with either drug. This would support an idea of different mechanisms for psychosis in BP-1 and SZ. The question posed here is not currently answered. This will also become interesting in the area of SZ therapeutics when effective cognitive enhancers are available. Then we will be able to distinguish whether APDs influence cognitive dysfunction to some degree in SZ or only psychosis, and vice versa.

Problems With Dimensional Treatments and the Weakness of Domain Diagnosis

The proposal to treat diseases by dimensions rather than by traditional diagnosis implies that there is more than one independent component to an illness. Therefore, the "rational" treatment would be done with more than one targeted treatment, individualized to a domain. One problem with this approach to therapeutics is that *it encourages polypharmacy.* Studies of medication administered in actual psychiatric practice indicate that there are already substantial degrees of polypharmacy. The use of polypharmacy can only rarely be supported by controlled clinical trials. Many clinical scientists are critical of polypharmacy. Patients may be kept on drugs because the physician is not certain that there is no clinical benefit. It is often unclear which medications help and which do not, without highly systematized follow-up. Controlled studies are important to guide clinician practice. In lieu of these kinds of data, recording the presence or absence of benefits of a new drug for a particular patient is particularly important in clinical practice. Each physician needs to be committed to discontinuing medications that are not beneficial. Testing the discontinuation of existing medications will help clarify for an individual person whether combined treatment is more useful than a core single treatment.

In general medicine, several disease entities can produce impairment in a psychophysiological process common to these entities. For example, infectious diseases and autoimmune diseases both produce fever; many etiologies produce arrhythmias. In a more general sense, the strategy of breaking down phenomena into different dimension has been used by a wide variety of sciences and is commonly used in psychology. At the present time, however, there *is not full agreement* as to how to subclassify schizophrenic or bipolar patients into categories or into meaningful dimensions. Drug response within either subcategories or dimensions has not been uniformly studied. The action of APDs in the psychosis domain of SZ or BP-1 is an example where this has been established, yet not with the diagnostic groups together. Also, it is difficult to be precise about similarities or differences because assessments are made with different instruments. A dimensional approach to psychopathology can be useful in diagnostic nomenclatures and in research, where they are specifically defined and studied in parallel. For example, if mania had been classified as psychotic versus nonpsychotic when lithium was initially tested, this information could have been obtained from early clinical trials. Then, we would already know whether lithium is effective in the psychotic component of mania.

There is *insufficient research* to definitively answer questions of the usefulness of dimensional classification even between SZ and BP-1. A common rating scale for use across diagnoses in rating the dimension of psychosis has not been critically developed, nor has it been applied to tracking clinical improvement during drug treatment in the psychosis dimension of different diagnoses. The development and use of assessment methodologies as well as the support of actual trials using dimensional classifications would facilitate the gathering of data to answer dimensional questions. In this book, the implications of various domains of psychiatric research for the diagnosis of mania and BD and their subtypes are presented. It would be of interest and potentially clinically important if one of these subtypes or dimensions identified patients who may have a differentially better clinical response to antipsychotic medicines or a subclass of antipsychotic medicines. In order for this research to elucidate these relationships, it is necessary 1) to identify a dimension or subtype, 2) to assess it in patients of diverse diagnoses in a clinical trial, and 3) to measure the difference in response either in global improvement or on specific dimensions. This could lead to a conclusion that targeting patients with the psychosis dimension with a given treatment will lead to a distinctive outcome.

Putative Mechanisms of APD Action

It is important to evaluate the possibility posed earlier in this chapter that similar drug responsiveness within a multidiagnosis dimension (if this could be rigorously demonstrated) might signal a common pathophysiology for psychosis. Evidence rather convincingly suggests that antipsychotic actions are effected through D_2 dopamine receptor blockade.[63,64] However, the functional mechanisms whereby that D_2 dopamine receptor blockade translates into an antipsychotic action in SZ or BD has not been fully defined. Moreover, establishing the mechanism for antipsychotic effects across different psychotic diagnoses would be informative no matter what the outcome. If similar regions and pathways of action were demonstrated, it would strengthen the explanation of mechanism. If differences in these parameters were found, it would provide more opportunity for the study of cerebral mechanisms.

Biomarkers of APD actions not only mark drug effects but also can contribute to an understanding of disease mechanisms. In the case of the discussion of the commonality of psychosis dimensions, biomarkers can also help define which illness characteristics belong to a biological entity. The use of biomarkers has already been applied in psychiatric genetic studies and can be a model in this regard. The association of specific genes with psychiatric diagnoses has been not as robust as hoped. Therefore, scientists have proceeded to use what Gottesman and Gould call "endophenotypic" characteristics of the illness to associate with genetic markers.[65] These are reflections of brain function close to its biology. Hence, they include characteristics of eye movements, evoked potential responses to sensory stimuli, estimates of sensory gating, and brain volume and functional characteristics of brain response. These measures of genetics, human brain imaging, molecular analysis of postmortem tissue, electrophysiology, and startle have already been applied to diagnoses but not yet applied to understanding the dimensional borders within diagnoses. Across SZ and BP-1, data show that several genes associate with both diagnoses (e.g., *NRG1, BDNF, DISC, G72/DAAO*), while some associate specifically with SZ (e.g., dysbindin, *COMT*, and *RGS4*) and others specifically with BD (e.g., Clock, *BMAL1,* and Period). Brain volume characteristics of BP-1 with psychosis are more like SZ than like nonpsychotic BD, but still distinctive in some respects from SZ. The use of these kinds of biomarkers to examine the domain of psychosis across diagnoses would be valuable in pursuing these questions about domain biology.

We have previously studied the pathways of functional antipsychotic action in human SZ volunteers using in vivo functional brain imaging to define brain regions affected by APDs.[66] In this study, 12 volunteers with SZ were given haloperidol or placebo, each compound for 1 month in random order; a positron emission tomography (PET) scan using fluorodeoxyglucose was carried out at the end of each month. The resulting data set included 12 sets of within-subject, functional imaging PET scans after haloperidol or placebo. The analysis showed an increase in neuronal activity (as indicated by an increase in glucose utilization) in the basal ganglia when the volunteers were taking haloperidol, both in caudate and putamen, as expected. It also showed that the APD increases glucose utilization in the anterior thalamus and decreases activity in the dorsolateral prefrontal cortex (DLPFC) and in the anterior cingulate cortex (ACC) (Figure 11–1). Because these regions represent areas important to the cortico-striato-thalamic pathways already well defined for motor function,[67] it was most parsimonious to make the interpretation that APDs use the brain's own long-tract neuronal pathways to project the effects of D_2 dopamine receptor blockade from the basal ganglia through the thalamus to the anterior aspects of the neocortex, particularly to the DLPFC and to the ACC (Figure 11–2). Our studies comparing first- and second-generation APDs in animals[68] lead us to postulate that both of these groups of APDs will act through this pathway, but the SGAs will be more selective regionally within the striatum in targeting the ventral striatum; this will lead to a more selective activation/inhibition within the long-track pathways and eventually to a more selective action in the cortical target regions. Also, the SGAs will exert additional actions directly in cortex because of the plethora there of 5-HT$_2$ serotonin receptors.[69] However, the effects of SGAs remain to be fully demonstrated in humans.

The example detailed above illustrates the use of a translational methodology applied to the understanding of antipsychotic actions of APDs in SZ. Had we used this approach across diagnostic classes (e.g., in SZ and BP-1), we could comment on the similarities and dissimilarities of APD actions in these different diagnoses. However, the above patient group included only volunteers with schizophrenic psychosis. In a test of dimensional versus diagnostic approaches, one could examine different diagnostic groups with functional brain imaging in their response to

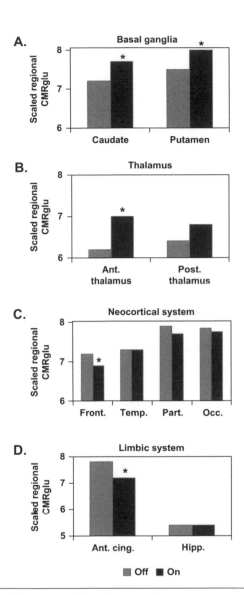

FIGURE 11–1. Positron emission tomography scans were acquired in 12 volunteers with schizophrenia using fluorodeoxyglucose after a 30-day treatment period with haloperidol (0.3 mg/kg/day) and with placebo.[65]

Cerebral metabolic rate for glucose utilization (CMRglu) was calculated regionally. With haloperidol treatment, the CMRglu was increased in basal ganglia *(caudate and putamen)* and in the anterior part of the thalamus *(ant. thalamus)*. CMRglu was decreased in the frontal cortex *(front.)* and in the anterior cingulate cortex *(ant. cing.)*.

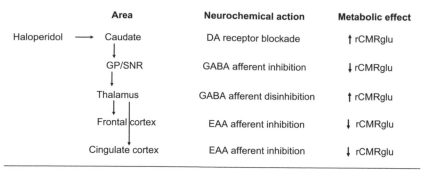

	Area	Neurochemical action	Metabolic effect
Haloperidol →	Caudate	DA receptor blockade	↑ rCMRglu
	GP/SNR	GABA afferent inhibition	↓ rCMRglu
	Thalamus	GABA afferent disinhibition	↑ rCMRglu
	Frontal cortex	EAA afferent inhibition	↓ rCMRglu
	Cingulate cortex	EAA afferent inhibition	↓ rCMRglu

FIGURE 11–2.   Basal ganglia–thalamic–cortical circuit: pathway of haloperidol-induced effects.

DA=dopamine; EAA=excitatory amino acid; GABA=γ-aminobutyric acid; GP/SNR=globus pallidus/substantia nigra pars reticulata; rCMRglu=regional cerebral metabolic rate for glucose utilization.

We used the data from Figure 11–1 to develop a hypothesis regarding the pathways associated with antipsychotic drug response. We suggest that the effect of haloperidol is initially exerted in the basal ganglia, then "projected" through the brain's own pathways first to the anterior thalamus, then up to the prefrontal cortex, both to the dorsolateral prefrontal cortex and to the anterior cingulate cortex, thus modulating brain activity throughout the cortico-striato-thalamic system.

the same APD treatments. This experiment would recruit people with psychosis and different diagnoses according to an a priori definition and study them in a parallel manner. This would include using a cross-diagnosis, validated psychosis rating scale, following treatment response across diagnoses and correlating treatment response with functional imaging data in all volunteers. Such a study would characterize the antipsychotic response across diagnostic groups. The approach would provide answers to questions of commonality of antipsychotic mechanisms across diagnostic groups. Moreover, it would rely on validated psychosis rating scales for marking psychosis response. Ideally, such comparative studies would also include other biomarkers, like electrophysiological characteristics, brain regional volumes, eye movement paradigms, and neuropsychological measures, all of which are used to characterize "endophenotypes" across diagnoses.[65]

The task of defining and validating a common psychosis dimension across diagnostic boundaries will need to include clinical, epidemiological, phenotypic, imaging, and molecular evidence as well as the pharmacological data we have presented here. The strength of the current DSM diagnostic system for mental disorders is its reliability, not its validity, the latter being still unknown for most psychiatric diagnoses.[3] One consideration is whether we will need to use additional "bining" systems in order to identify valid molecular characteristics of mental conditions or if dimensional definitions will improve the detection of etiological and pathophysiological mechanisms.[70] Brain and symptom response to pharmacological agents, especially APDs, will be an important aspect of this examination.

It is the development of data sets like the one proposed above that would begin to give us some information about the biology of antipsychotic response across diagnostic groups and help us verify (or not) dimensional concepts of psychosis, as suggested, but not demonstrated, in the literature. Overall, even when tested with pharmacology, the data are inadequate to rigorously demonstrate that psychosis across SZ and BD is the same construct. As psychiatry gradually gains information about the altered brain mechanisms in its illnesses, diagnoses will be resorted, based on firm knowledge of pathophysiology. Nonetheless, asking questions of diagnoses provides obvious pathways to studies that will contribute to defining pathophysiology.

Summary: Using Pharmacology to Define Psychosis as a Dimension That Crosses Diagnostic Boundaries

This chapter reviews the clinical treatment response data in SZ and BP-1. Based on these data, we can say that the psychosis domain of both diagnoses responds therapeutically to APDs. Yet this commonality of response has not been examined side-by-side in the same study. Therefore, the phenomenology of the psychosis, the course of response, and the pharmacology across APDs of the treatment response still has to be characterized. The use of pharmacological approaches to examine the dimension of psychosis across diagnoses is highly indicated and could be done. The characterization of treatment response to APDs would be most valuable in the context of a broader phenotyping effort in an attempt to use clinical genetic methodologies to define dimensional borders within and across diagnoses.

References

1. American Psychiatric Association. Diagnostic and Statistical Manual of Mental Disorders. 4th ed. Washington, DC: American Psychiatric Association; 1994.
2. Gardner DM, Baldessarini RJ, Waraich P. Modern antipsychotic drugs: a critical overview. CMAJ. 2005;172:1703–1711.
3. Hyman SE, Fenton WS. Medicine: what are the right targets for psychopharmacology? Science. 2003;299:350–351.
4. Marder SR, Fenton W. Measurement and treatment research to improve cognition in schizophrenia: NIMH MATRICS initiative to support the development of agents for improving cognition in schizophrenia. Schizophr Res. 2004;72:5–9.
5. Carpenter WT Jr, Buchanan RW. Schizophrenia [review]. N Engl J Med. 1994;330:681–690.

6. Tamminga CA. Principles of the pharmacotherapy of schizophrenia. In: Charney DS, Nestler EJ, eds. Neurobiology of Mental Illness. New York: Oxford University Press; 1999:272–285.

7. American Psychiatric Association. Practice guideline for the treatment of patients with schizophrenia. Am J Psychiatry. 1997;154:1–63.

8. Davis JM, Chen N. Dose response and dose equivalence of antipsychotics. [see comment]. J Clin Psychopharmacol. 2004;24:192–208.

9. Davis JM. Review of antipsychotic drug literature. In: Klein DF, Davis JM, eds. Diagnosis and Drug Treatment of Psychiatric Disorders. Baltimore, MD: Williams and Wilkins; 1969:52–138.

10. Davis JM, Chen N, Glick ID. A meta-analysis of the efficacy of second-generation antipsychotics. [see comment]. Arch Gen Psychiatry. 2003;60:553–564.

11. Leucht S, Pitschel-Walz G, Abraham D, Kissling W. Efficacy and extrapyramidal side-effects of the new antipsychotics olanzapine, quetiapine, risperidone, and sertindole compared to conventional antipsychotics and placebo. A meta-analysis of randomized controlled trials. Schizophr Res. 1999;35:51–68.

12. Leucht S, Pitschel-Walz G, Engel RR, Kissling W. Amisulpride, an unusual "atypical" antipsychotic: a meta-analysis of randomized controlled trials. [see comment]. Am J Psychiatry. 2002;159:180–190.

13. Leucht S, Wahlbeck K, Hamann J, Kissling W. New generation antipsychotics versus low-potency conventional antipsychotics: a systematic review and meta-analysis. [see comment]. Lancet. 2003;361:1581–1589.

14. Wahlbeck K, Cheine M, Essali A, Adams C. Evidence of clozapine's effectiveness in schizophrenia: a systematic review and meta-analysis of randomized trials. Am J Psychiatry. 1999;156:990–999.

15. Lieberman JA, Stroup TS, McEvoy JP, et al. Effectiveness of antipsychotic drugs in patients with chronic schizophrenia. N Engl J Med. 2005;353:1209–1223.

16. McEvoy JP, Lieberman JA, Stroup TS, et al. Effectiveness of clozapine versus olanzapine, quetiapine, and risperidone in patients with chronic schizophrenia who did not respond to prior atypical antipsychotic treatment. Am J Psychiatry. 2006;163:600–610.

17. Stroup TS, Lieberman JA, McEvoy JP, et al. Effectiveness of olanzapine, quetiapine, risperidone, and ziprasidone in patients with chronic schizophrenia following discontinuation of a previous atypical antipsychotic. Am J Psychiatry. 2006;163:611–622.

18. Marder SR, McQuade RD, Stock E, et al. Aripiprazole in the treatment of schizophrenia: safety and tolerability in short-term, placebo-controlled trials. Schizophr Res. 2003;61:123–136.

19. Tandon R, Marcus RN, Stock EG, et al. A prospective, multicenter, randomized, parallel-group, open-label study of aripiprazole in the management of patients with schizophrenia or schizoaffective disorder in general psychiatric practice: Broad Effectiveness Trial With Aripiprazole (BETA). Schizophr Res. 2006;84:77–89.

20. Kasper S, Lerman MN, McQuade RD, et al. Efficacy and safety of aripiprazole vs. haloperidol for long-term maintenance treatment following acute relapse of schizophrenia. Int J Neuropsychopharmacol. 2003;6:325–337.

21. Kane JM, Carson WH, Saha AR, et al. Efficacy and safety of aripiprazole and haloperidol versus placebo in patients with schizophrenia and schizoaffective disorder. J Clin Psychiatry. 2002;63:763–771.
22. El-Sayeh HG, Morganti C. Aripiprazole for schizophrenia. Cochrane Database Syst Rev. 2006;CD004578.
23. Wlodzimierz KC, Ronald NM, Anne T, Margaretta N, Robert DM. Effectiveness of long-term aripiprazole therapy in patients with acutely relapsing or chronic, stable schizophrenia: a 52-week, open-label comparison with olanzapine. Psychopharmacology. 2006;189:259–266.
24. Buchanan RW, Kirkpatrick B, Summerfelt A, Hanlon TE, Levine J, Carpenter WT. Clinical predictors of relapse following neuroleptic withdrawal. Biol Psychiatry. 1992;32:72–78.
25. Lieberman JA, Kane JM, Gadaleta D, Brenner R, Lesser MS, Kinon B. Methylphenidate challenge as a predictor of relapse in schizophrenia. Am J Psychiatry. 1984;41:633–638.
26. Ventura J, Nuechterlein KH, Hardesty JP, Gitlin M. Life events and schizophrenic relapse after withdrawal of medication. Br J Psychiatry. 1992;161:615–620.
27. Ghaemi SN. New treatments for bipolar disorder: the role of atypical neuroleptic agents. J Clin Psychiatry. 2000;61(suppl 14):33–42.
28. Keefe RSE, Young CA, Rock SL, Purdon SE, Gold JM, Breier A. One-year double-blind study of the neurocognitive efficacy of olanzapine, risperidone, and haloperidol in schizophrenia. Schizophr Res. 2006;81:1–15.
29. Harvey PD, Patterson TL, Potter LS, Zhong K, Brecher M. Improvement in social competence with short-term atypical antipsychotic treatment: a randomized, double-blind comparison of quetiapine versus risperidone for social competence, social cognition, and neuropsychological functioning. Am J Psychiatry. 2006;163:1918–1925.
30. Kane J, Honigfeld G, Singer J, Meltzer H. Clozapine for the treatment-resistant schizophrenic. A double-blind comparison with chlorpromazine. Arch Gen Psychiatry. 1988;45:789–796.
31. Glick ID, Pham D, Davis JM. Concomitant medications may not improve outcome of antipsychotic monotherapy for stabilized patients with nonacute schizophrenia. J Clin Psychiatry. 2006;67:1261–1265.
32. Dunner DL. Safety and tolerability of emerging pharmacological treatments for bipolar disorder. Bipolar Disord. 2005;7:307–325.
33. Ehret MJ, Levin GM. Long-term use of atypical antipsychotics in bipolar disorder. Pharmacotherapy. 2006;26:1134–1147.
34. Gajwani P, Kemp DE, Muzina DJ, Xia G, Gao K, Calabrese JR. Acute treatment of mania: an update on new medications. Curr Psychiatry Rep. 2006;8:504–509.
35. Scherk MD, Pajonk FG, Leucht S. Second-generation antipsychotic agents in the treatment of acute mania. Arch Gen Psychiatry. 2007;64:442–455.
36. Seemuller F, Forsthoff A, Dittmann S, et al. The safety and tolerability of atypical antipsychotics in bipolar disorder. Expert Opin Drug Saf. 2005;4:849–868.
37. Newcomer JW. Medical risk in patients with bipolar disorder and schizophrenia. J Clin Psychiatry. 2006;67:e16.

38. McElroy SL, Keck PE. Pharmacologic agents for the treatment of acute bipolar mania. Biol Psychiatry. 2000;48:539–557.

39. Dunner DL. Atypical antipsychotics: efficacy across bipolar disorder subpopulations. J Clin Psychiatry. 2005;66(suppl 3):20–27.

40. McIntyre RS, Konarski JZ. Tolerability profiles of atypical antipsychotics in the treatment of bipolar disorder. J Clin Psychiatry. 2005;66:28–36.

41. Kane JM. Tardive dyskinesia in affective disorders. J Clin Psychiatry. 1999;60(suppl 5):43–47.

42. Craig TJ, Grossman S, Mojtabai R, et al. Medication use patterns and 2-year outcome in first-admission bipolar disorder with psychotic features. Bipolar Disord. 2004;6:406–415.

43. Bowden CL, Swann AC, Calabrese JR, et al. A randomized, placebo-controlled, multicenter study of divalproex sodium extended release in the treatment of acute mania. J Clin Psychiatry. 2006;67:1501–1510.

44. Oral TE. Treatment of acute mania. Neuro Endocrinol Lett. 2005;26:9–25.

45. Tohen M, Strakowski SM, Zarate C, et al. The McLean-Harvard first-episode project: 6-month symptomatic and functional outcome in affective and nonaffective psychosis. Biol Psychiatry. 2000;48:467–476.

46. Schatzberg AF. Employing pharmacologic treatment of bipolar disorder to greatest effect. J Clin Psychiatry. 2004;65:15–20.

47. Marken PA, Pies RW. Emerging treatments for bipolar disorder: safety and adverse effect profiles. Ann Pharmacother. 2006;40:276–285

48. Klein DF, Davis JM. Diagnosis and Drug Treatment of Psychiatric Disorders. Baltimore, MD: Williams and Wilkins; 1969.

49. Calabrese JR, Goldberg JF, Ketter TA, et al. Recurrence in bipolar I disorder: a post hoc analysis excluding relapses in two double-blind maintenance studies. Biol Psychiatry. 2006;59:1061–1064.

50. Keck PE Jr, Calabrese JR, McQuade RD, et al. A randomized, double-blind, placebo-controlled 26-week trial of aripiprazole in recently manic patients with bipolar I disorder. J Clin Psychiatry. 2006;67:626–637.

51. Davis JM. Overview: maintenance therapy in psychiatry: II. Affective disorders. Am J Psychiatry. 1976;133:1–13.

52. Davis JM. Chapter 10: Lithium Maintenance of Unipolar Depression. In: Bauer M, ed. Lithium in Neuropsychiatry: The Comprehensive Guide. Abingdon, Oxon, England: Informa UK; 2006:99–108.

53. Baldessarini RJ, Tondo L, Davis P, Pompili M, Goodwin FK, Hennen J. Decreased risk of suicides and attempts during long-term lithium treatment: a meta-analytic review. Bipolar Disord. 2006;8:625–639.

54. Tohen M, Chengappa KN, Suppes T, et al. Relapse prevention in bipolar I disorder: 18-month comparison of olanzapine plus mood stabiliser v. mood stabiliser alone. Br J Psychiatry. 2004;184:337–345.

55. Tohen M, Ketter TA, Zarate CA, et al. Olanzapine versus divalproex sodium for the treatment of acute mania and maintenance of remission: a 47-week study. Am J Psychiatry. 2003;160:1263–1271.

56. Bowden CL. Atypical antipsychotic augmentation of mood stabilizer therapy in bipolar disorder. J Clin Psychiatry. 2005;66(suppl 3):12–19.

57. Bowden CL. Treatment options for bipolar depression. J Clin Psychiatry. 2005;66(suppl 1):3–6.

58. Calabrese JR, Keck PE Jr, Macfadden W, et al. A randomized, double-blind, placebo-controlled trial of quetiapine in the treatment of bipolar I or II depression. Am J Psychiatry. 2005;162:1351–1360.

59. Gao K, Calabrese JR. Newer treatment studies for bipolar depression. Bipolar Disord. 2005;7(suppl 5):13–23.

60. Gao K, Gajwani P, Elhaj O, Calabrese JR. Typical and atypical antipsychotics in bipolar depression. J Clin Psychiatry. 2005;66:1376–1385.

61. Thase ME, Macfadden W, Weisler RH, et al. Efficacy of quetiapine monotherapy in bipolar I and II depression: a double-blind, placebo-controlled study (the BOLDER II study). J Clin Psychopharmacol. 2006;26:600–609.

62. Pande AC, Crockatt JG, Janney CA, Werth JL, Tsaroucha G. Gabapentin in bipolar disorder: a placebo-controlled trial of adjunctive therapy. Gabapentin Bipolar Disorder Study Group. Bipolar Disord. 2000;2:249–255.

63. Carlsson A, Lindquist L. Effect of chlorpromazine or haloperidol on formation of 3-methoxytyramine and normetanephrine in mouse brain. Acta Pharmacol Toxicol. 1963;20:140–145.

64. Seeman P, Van Tol HH. Dopamine receptor pharmacology. Trends Pharmacol Sci. 1994;15:264–270.

65. Gottesman II, Gould T. The endophenotype concept in psychiatry: etymology and strategic intentions. Am J Psychiatry. 2003;160:636–645.

66. Holcomb HH, Cascella NG, Thaker GK, Medoff DR, Dannals RF, Tamminga CA. Functional sites of neuroleptic drug action in the human brain: PET/FDG studies with and without haloperidol. Am J Psychiatry. 1996;153:41–49.

67. DeLong MR. Primate models of movement disorders of basal ganglia origin [Review]. Trends Neurosci. 1990;13:281–285.

68. Shirakawa O, Tamminga CA. Basal ganglia GABAA and dopamine D1 binding site correlates of haloperidol-induced oral dyskinesias in rat. Exp Neurol. 1994;127:62–69.

69. Bymaster FP, Rasmussen K, Calligaro DO, et al. In vitro and in vivo biochemistry of olanzapine: a novel, atypical antipsychotic drug. J Clin Psychiatry. 1997;58:28–36.

70. Carpenter WT Jr, Buchanan RW, Kirkpatrick B, Tamminga C, Wood F. Strong inference, theory testing, and the neuroanatomy of schizophrenia. Arch Gen Psychiatry. 1993;50:825–831.

INDEX

Page numbers printed in **boldface** *type refer to tables or figures.*